POWER TOOLS - THE ULTIMATE OWNER'S MANUAL FOR PERSONAL EMPOWERMENT

As an ex-building con' [barcode] .annel of spirit, a book of spiritual P [barcode] .r my hot buttons. I clearly remember t. [barcode] an electric screw driver. My first thought wa. [barcode] .fe just got easier and my second thought was how . ime and energy I had wasted in the past. In this book Jean shows us a practical approach to true empowerment and gives the details needed to use the new tools of empowerment.

Steve Rother – Spokesman for the group, Author, and Host of the VirtualLight Broadcast at Lightworker.com

Jean Adrienne has taken the most important key in creation-YOU-and mapped out a glorious, joyful, and easy way to access your true power and authenticity. You will shift your Knowing with this book. I did.

Dee Wallace – Actor, Author, Healer. www.IAMDeeWallace.com

Everyone knows you can't build a house with cookie dough and a spatula, yet so many people think they can build the lives they want with goo and a fork. In her new book, Jean gives you the tools to not only break new ground, but build the palace you've always wanted to come home to.

Jarrad Hewett – Channel and Author of Love, Life, God: The Journey of Creation. www.JarradHewett.com

Conscious creation comes alive in very practical ways in this insightful book by Jean Adrienne. If you are new to the topic you will find this guide useful and simple to navigate. If you've been playing with manifestation for years you are bound to come away with deeper integration and a fresh perspective. Thank you for this gem!

Lisa Michaels – Author and President of Natural Rhythms. www.NaturalRhythms.org

Power Tools

The Ultimate Owner's Manual
for Personal Empowerment

Power Tools

The Ultimate Owner's Manual
for Personal Empowerment

Jean Adrienne

Winchester, UK
Washington, USA

First published by Soul Rocks Books, 2013
Soul Rocks Books is an imprint of John Hunt Publishing Ltd., Laurel House, Station Approach,
Alresford, Hants, SO24 9JH, UK
office1@jhpbooks.net
www.johnhuntpublishing.com
www.soulrocks-books.com

For distributor details and how to order please visit the 'Ordering' section on our website.

Text copyright: Jean Adrienne 2012

ISBN: 978 1 78099 519 9

A CIP catalogue record for this book is available from the British Library.

Design: Stuart Davies

Printed and bound by CPI Group (UK) Ltd, Croydon, CR0 4YY

We operate a distinctive and ethical publishing philosophy in all
areas of our business, from our global network of authors to
production and worldwide distribution.

CONTENTS

The Chambered Nautilus

This is the ship of pearl, which, poets feign,
Sails the unshadowed main, —
The venturous bark that flings
On the sweet summer wind its purpled wings
In gulfs enchanted, where the Siren sings,
And coral reefs lie bare,
Where the cold sea-maids rise to sun their streaming hair.

Its webs of living gauze no more unfurl;
Wrecked is the ship of pearl!
And every chambered cell,
Where its dim dreaming life was wont to dwell,
As the frail tenant shaped his growing shell,
Before thee lies revealed, —
Its irised ceiling rent, its sunless crypt unsealed!

Year after year beheld the silent toil
That spread his lustrous coil;
Still, as the spiral grew,
He left the past year's dwelling for the new,
Stole with soft step its shining archway through,
Built up its idle door,
Stretched in his last-found home, and knew the old no more.

Thanks for the heavenly message brought by thee,
Child of the wandering sea,
Cast from her lap, forlorn!
From thy dead lips a clearer note is born
Than ever Triton blew from wreathèd horn!
While on mine ear it rings,
Through the deep caves of thought I hear a voice that sings:

Build thee more stately mansions, O my soul,
As the swift seasons roll!
Leave thy low-vaulted past!
Let each new temple, nobler than the last,
Shut thee from heaven with a dome more vast,
Till thou at length art free,
Leaving thine outgrown shell by life's unresting sea!

by: Oliver Wendell Holmes (1809-1894)

Introduction

This morning I had an epiphany. It had to do with Power. Personal Power. I woke to the understanding of what that means in a flash of insight. For almost all of my life, I have played 'small'. I told myself I was just Jean. It never occurred to me to look at the other possibility—that I might actually be GREAT. Greatness was something that famous people were, folks who had invented something big or were elected to an office of great power or who were rock stars or actors—certainly not a girl from Tallahassee who had been married four times and raised two kids as a single mom and lived a middle-class existence...

Today I woke up to my Power. The wake-up call came in the form of an email from a man in Brazil who didn't understand something I had written. He wanted to know what it meant to 'stand in your power' because he said there didn't seem to be a direct translation for that in his language. The only way I could begin to explain it was to look at my own life to see what that phrase meant to me. That's when I got it! In that moment I realized who I was, what I had done, and how many lives I have touched. In that moment I was able to see my own greatness. That epiphany allowed me to look back over the last 63 years and realize that in actuality I was BORN great – that we all are. I clearly saw that over the next fifty years I then allowed myself to slip into mediocrity, in order to 'fit in', giving away that power that was my birth right to anyone who wanted it (and many who didn't!) Then a little over ten years ago, I began to wake up. I experienced a calling to do more than just get by. It started with writing, moved into listening and became full-fledged passion. That is what I want to share with you. The tools that help us to figure this out are all around us. On the surface they appear to be commonplace, but at a much deeper level they can help us to change our lives into so much more than we could have imagined.

Welcome to my workshop. I've cleaned and organized my tools so that you can find everything you need, and I am happy to let you borrow this space while you are settling into this 'Great Shift'. You are welcome to use all the materials as well so that you can build yourself a grand new reality. My workshop is your workshop! The only thing I ask is that you stay really present while you work, because these are power tools you will be using, after all.

This workshop has a unique power generation system—the frequency of love. Love is a vibration, outside the range of the human ear. It's a tone in the 16th harmonic, and it is the frequency of life, of creation. All the power tools in my shop plug into this generator, and the supply is unlimited, the cost is free.

We are in interesting times. Things are moving so quickly, and energy supports our creations. We are making things happen with our minds, and some of us are creating our worst nightmares without realizing it. We have no one to blame but ourselves. At other times we are creating our heart's desires without even trying. Our old pal, time lag, has gone on extended vacation. He used to save us when we thought those thoughts that had the potential to wreak havoc, and now either havoc or heaven waits for a crack in our mental space.

Interestingly enough, we come here, take on physicality and 'borrow' these bodies to live our lives and learn lessons that can only be learned this way, but we don't bring an owner's manual with us. It would appear we forgot to pack it in our bag of tricks! This book is designed to fill in the blanks as you become more and more awake and realize that perhaps you need a little guidance along the way.

We stand at the portal of a new reality. It has been prophesied for eons, with the most famous one being the Mayan calendar. Why would anyone want to miss out on every possible aspect of this great shift? Yet a huge percentage of the population of the planet is still sleepwalking, blissfully unaware of pure potential and completely convinced that they are the victims of 'the powers that be'. They have no clue that with a sudden change of mind, they could win the lottery!

Most of us would like to be able to manifest everything we want—like winning the lottery, new cars, the love of our life, etc. If we could figure out how to do it, we would already have it all. The "how" just seems to be outside our reach, and we get discouraged and give up. Personally, I got tired of haphazard creation. After studying metaphysics for many years, I knew that I was the only one making things happen in my life, so I reached a point where I was ready to take responsibility for it all—the good, the bad, the ugly. This commitment brought me a break-through. I opened to a new level of listening and a new category of experience. I had to find a new set of tools in order to make things happen when I wanted them to. And I had to learn how to use them, because the owner's manuals didn't always translate correctly. Some of the tools I found didn't even have manuals. So my first creation had to be this Owner's Manual.

There is a pattern in manifestation. There have always been directions for using our tools. They are actually quite clear, but until recently, I either didn't want to see them or was blind to them. The rules were always there, however, and looking back, I was able to realize that when I played by them I got what I wanted, and when I didn't, well… This information on Universal Laws and conscious creation has been brought to the forefront by many over the last twenty years, so I didn't want to write a book saying the same old, same old. My goal is to bring forward infor-mation to enable the reader to stand in the place of personal power and move onward and upward.

Each of us is being called to search for and strive for balance in our lives. We are being nudged, if not forced, to let go of everything that doesn't serve us anymore—everything that holds us back and keeps us stuck in duality. For some people this means the loss of a job, for others, the loss of a home, and for even others, the loss of a relationship, either through choice or, in some cases, a death. Because we have become conditioned to believe that change MEANS loss, a lot of us are looking at circumstances as exactly that, and not stopping to ponder that sometimes, always actually, these changes are moving us toward something better. Sometimes it's hard to see this through the tears. One of the tools we are going to use will be the Jack Hammer. What a great metaphor for digging in and breaking up the foundation of our reality so that we can build something architecturally phenomenal, where once we had a starter home.

It is for this reason that this book is being presented to you. It's a gift of power tools from my heart to assist us as we move through what many call 'precarious times'. Another way to look at them is as 'precious times' because I believe that we have more of an opportunity now than we have ever had before to let go of everything holding us back and go for the gold, the 'new reality', Heaven on Earth!

Another gift that is contained in this book is a set of messages from the Beings of NOW, Light energies from Source who are here to assist us in moving gracefully through these times of intense change while we move into higher consciousness. They are sharing tools to help us grow in consciousness. They provide their guidance at the beginning of each chapter. They have also shared their wisdom throughout the book to show us new ways of looking at multidimensionality and our own DNA.

DNA is amazing. It is multidimensional and quantum. It holds everything that ever was and everything that ever will be, and it allows each of us, as individuals, to choose how much—or how little we will allow in our lives. As you read, you will open to more possibilities than you might have allowed yourself to consider before.

As an introduction to the Beings of NOW, here is a recent message that will share their love, along with their sense of humor:

"Greetings Dear Ones. We are the Beings of NOW, and we are here to serve and assist you as you move through these wonderful times. These are times of new beginnings. They are times for the shift in your thinking that will also shift your creative process. It is time for opening yourselves to the larger field of potential, because the time for thinking small has passed. You have each glimpsed what life is like when you remove the barriers, and it felt good, did it not? We tell you that today these barriers are being dissolved, and the limitations you have had in the past are removed permanently. You can now allow your thought process to simply expand outward past where your beliefs had limited you in the past. Expand outward in ever increasing circles. You are now being allowed to be aware of your involvement in the creative process – you can now see the bigger picture of how it works.

It is a point we ponder as we try to understand human thought process. We simply find it difficult to see why you have perceived that there were limitations to begin with. We have been observing how you play with creativity, and in order to explain what we are meaning, we will use money as our example, because this is what gets your attention the fastest.

You want money, more money so you can do things you have always wanted to do; so you create a process to bring you money. You call it a job and it works for you because you intend this to be so – and conversely, you work for IT because energy has to flow. Are you with us so far? And you think, Oh – I can do every-thing I want to do if I can earn (hear it – EARN) only $2500 a week. Do you see how limiting this structure is? First, you limit how much you can experience by the amount you believe you deserve. Then you decide that you have to toil for the money in order to justify that you deserve it because you earned it!

We would assure you that this is all a game – a grand game that you created for yourself and one that you can stop playing anytime you choose to. It is a game and it truly has nothing to do with reality. We find this perplexing as we try to understand why you are so attached to your game!

We would now share with you another view that is much closer to the truth. There are no limits to what you can have, be, do, experience. You do not have to DO anything in order to receive. You just have to BE. It seems almost too simple, doesn't it? You crafted your game because you just didn't think it would be that easy – and because you believed this to be true... Well, we think you are getting the picture.

So, take a break from the game please. Just for today—try it our way. OK? For a moment, imagine all the possibilities you can—get outside your preconceived ideas and limits. Proceed with life knowing that you have all these things already, and watch how they materialize for you, one by one by one. Now begin to fill the space between your thoughts with abundance – abundant wealth, perfect health, abundant love, more success than you ever dreamed possible.

Energy builds upon energy. This is how the law of attraction works. As you begin to hold the frequency of love (which is the frequency of all of creation, you know) it acts like a magnet attracting to you more of the same frequency. So many of the things you hold dear or desire vibrate at the frequency of Divine love. We are talking about money, success, love and great health, remember—they are all reflections of this energy of Divine love. And as you become it, the energy begins to snowball and these reflections begin to amass. They grow geometrically according to the mathematical algorithm you call the Golden Mean Spiral. How many of you have heard the metaphor, 'the rich just keep getting richer?' Did you ever wonder why this was, and why you were stuck NOT getting richer? We have just solved this mystery for you. It begins with a single acceptance of a synchronicity, one bit of gratitude, which attracts another. The Golden Mean algorithm is the sum of each number added to the one previous.

So 1 + 1 = 2, 2 + 1 = 3, 3 + 2 = 5, 5 + 3 = 8, 8 + 5 = 13, 13 + 8 = 21, 21 + 13 = 34, and it goes on and on through infinity. Do you see how quickly it adds up? You would call it growing by leaps and bounds! And soon you have abundance in every area of your life. This is your birth right. It is truth and it is how the Universe works. Always.

Now let's look at how you create the negative stuff you deal with. It happens the same way, because the Universe works according to the same laws. Always. So, one negative thought, word or judgment begets another, then becomes 3, 5, 8, 13, 21, 34 and on and on.

All you have to do is remember this and you will be able to release the other stories and illusions. Just open your heart to receive. Become love. We know you are.

Enjoy!"

Chapter One

Why Me? Why You?

Why NOT you? Many of you have forgotten the choices you made prior to coming to Planet Earth. Our job is to remind you that it was a BIG decision on your part—certainly not an accident.

Why would you pick up this book today? There are no accidents, so there must be a reason. Have you heard enough already about 2012, ascension, yada yada? I know I had! It seemed like every day I would get a new 'forward' in my email with someone else telling me that the sky is falling, banks are crashing, the poles are shifting and California and Florida are about to return to the sea. Enough already!

Twenty years ago it wouldn't have mattered. I was completely bound by my old belief systems, based in fundamentalist Christianity. I didn't believe in reincarnation, karma and had never heard of such stuff as Universal Laws. I knew the Ten Commandments and the Golden Rule. I did my darndest to follow them, but being human, I screwed up a lot. Somewhere along the way I began to wake up. This nagging little voice kept telling me that I didn't have the whole story, that there was more, but I had no idea where to look. I started with the foundation I already had and completed a four year course of study through my church, but that didn't satisfy my yearning for the elusive truth. I stumbled upon metaphysics and energy medicine and spent the next ten years absorbing everything I could get my hands on. I really thought I had found it.

During all this time I continued my career in high-tech sales. I was good at selling and made a bunch of money, but it wasn't my passion. I might have found the truth, but I hadn't found my passion. (Now I realize I hadn't found my truth either!) I gleaned a great deal of experience in the corporate world—enough to show me things weren't working. At a deep level I knew there needed to be balance and that unless everybody wins, nobody wins, but this is not what I saw in my dealings in that world. As I began to spend more time looking inside, this dichotomy grew. It became more difficult every day to be one person at my job and another person in my spiritual life. Finally, I couldn't do it anymore. I began to devote more time to the things that were making me happy, even if they weren't the tasks that were paying the bills. I started writing—four books already and two decks of cards. I created a healing tool, InnerSpeak, and began to teach others how to use it in addition to facilitating healing sessions for clients and myself in my spare time. I was set free from a loveless marriage. I found Internet Talk Radio, started a show on consciousness, and met a ton of brilliant people who all had something to share. And I began to listen. I learned how to hear the voice of my Higher Self, my Angels and my teachers. Through this I began to create more.

One day I realized that assisting others to find their passion had become MY passion. At this point it was as though I had broken through a gigantic wall. I stepped into the flow instead of attempting (unsuccessfully) to row my boat upstream. Going with the flow is actually the only way we can be happy, but nobody ever told me that. I spent sixty years in the misconception that hard work and financial security was going to be the key to everything. So, nothing changed from the point of outward appearances. I still have my house and my car, still wear the same clothes and get my hair done at the same place, but actually, everything has changed. A shift has taken place in my perspective, and nothing will ever be the same again.

I invite you to share in my experiences, read about the lessons I have learned, and take what you want—leave the rest! As you work in my workshop, you will learn how to use the Jack Hammer to bust up the reality that doesn't serve you any more, the Compass and Square to define your boundaries and your truth, the Drill to anchor your new foundation, and the Framer to frame out the walls and define your space. You will get proficient using your Saw and Level, you will create a perfect blueprint for your construction project, and you will be amazed at what a grand architect you always were. The Magnet will attract your desires and assist you to receive and accept them. At the conclusion of this journey, you will be amazed at how far you have come when you step into the life you have created for yourself going forward. You will see what a fabulous building you have created from your own mind.

Chapter Two

Jack Hammer

The first word that comes to mind is strength. Your foundational
strength lies in your heart, in your ability to remain centered there
at all times. As you make decisions from your heart, they will
always come from the highest possible frequency and will serve the
good of all.

If we really want to make headway in our move toward higher
consciousness, we have to start from the bottom up. We have to
be committed to being here. Most of us spend considerably less
than 100% of each day in our bodies. Disassociation has become
a pandemic—the perfect coping tool in a hectic society where we
all have SO many commitments. We've forgotten what it means
to be grounded, and this leaves no stability to our energy. Our
first tool is required to create the foundation that will allow us to
live comfortably in our bodies and fully present on this planet.

How strong is your foundation? Unless it was prepared
properly, you can't expect your life to be stable. How involved
were you in the laying of that foundation anyway? Most of us
weren't involved at all. The edifice that is our reality was
probably constructed on the belief systems of others. Mine was—
and I bet yours was too. It's been an OK place to live until
recently, but I have outgrown mine, and every day I find areas
where my foundation is crumbling. I think it's time to start from
scratch—tear down the old and build it up right this time. Unless
the foundation is laid properly, the building will not pass
inspection. Why would you want to put so much work into such
a large project unless you were sure it would be stable and
strong?

The perfect tool for this is the Jack Hammer. It's noisy but efficient as it chops up the old beliefs that have turned to cement under our feet. Leave nothing. This time you will be designing and building your being on only solid beliefs. You will dig the foundation deep and pour the footings yourself, making sure that your reality is fully grounded.

What does grounding mean and how can it be accomplished? For many people, grounding is an electrical term meaning using the earth to complete a circuit. Take lightning, for example. Lightning is electrical energy in the sky that manifests as light. It is harmless and beautiful until it comes into contact with something that connects it to the earth. It is pure potential until it is grounded, and only then does its power become apparent. Therefore, if you look at your thoughts as lightning, they are magnificent, but merely potential until they become grounded unto reality. The goal of grounding, then, is to take each thought we want to consciously create and give it a path to earth, to this present reality.

How can you do this? If you can consider your physical body to be the conduit, it becomes easier to understand this process. First you conceive an idea in your mind. You pull it into your own field from the field of pure potential that is the Divine mind or universal consciousness. Imagine this idea flowing into you from your Higher Self and entering through your crown chakra on the top of your head. Now look at your spine as the lightning rod connecting your energy centers with the earth. Envision your idea flowing down your spine and out into the ground through the soles of your feet—actually it helps if you see yourself connected deep into the earth by roots that stretch out from your body and extend deep into the core of the planet. As your ideas are grounded, they become like seeds planted by the dark of the moon. Fertilize and water them with love, but leave them alone to grow. It doesn't help a flower to mature any faster if you tug on the sprout. That will just kill it. Everything blossoms when the time is right.

The difficulty most of us have is getting past the chaos in our heads. We have thousands of thoughts every moment. Grounding involves selective thinking... Choosing the ideas that are viable in the moment and sending only those to be planted — releasing the rest. This process of selecting is what enables our focus to be precise and generate the results we desire rather than those we don't.

As we move into higher consciousness selectivity becomes more and more important. We are spiritual beings having a human experience. Plant your feet firmly and extend your roots deeply, if you want to will allow your dreams to manifest into reality.

Now that you have released all the old belief systems that really weren't working for you before and cleared away the rubble, you are ready to develop a plan. So let's look in general at what kind of structure you want to create—a home, an office, a recreational facility, a high rise? Now is the time to really think about what you want in your life. Do you have a budget? Only if you believe you do, because budget is another one of those limiting belief systems, and you look like a no-limits kind of builder to me!

Choice and Focus Exercise

Draw a circle and divide it into six pie-shaped wedges. Label each one with the following classifications: Spirituality, Love, Friends, Exercise, Play and Work. Now place a dot in each pie wedge to show how much energy you place into each of these areas in your life today. A dot near the center of the circle indicates very little energy. A dot near the outer rim shows a lot of energy. Connect the dots. You can't begin to live in consciousness until you are fully aware where you are spending your time, your thinking and your energy. Keep this chart and update it as you feel yourself shifting into conscious living. As your priorities change and your time becomes more balanced, you might find that your "wheel of life" becomes better rounded, and that life lows more smoothly for you.

There is an additional challenge we face relative to grounding as we move further into this 'shift of the ages'. Our planet is changing as well. Her magnetic fields are becoming very fluid. This creates opportunities as we try to stay in sync with the magnetic pull of Earth. At times we feel genuinely disconnected because of these fluctuations. We've always taken gravity for granted, like death and taxes, but with these variations, our inner selves are thrown out of balance, and it is frightening. Because we are unaware of what's really happening, we might think we are ill or even a little crazy. It's important for each of us to renegotiate our relationship with gravity on a daily basis, consciously. The more attention we place on being connected to the Earth, to nature and to our physical bodies, the easier coming years will be. Who knows—gravity may never return to providing the stability it once did. Perhaps that job is up to us now!

Here is where you have to dig the footings deep. They have to be strong, and they have to be constructed from all the correct materials. For your project, I suggest that the footings be the four elements—earth, air, fire and water. Individually, they each bring a unique gift to our world, and together they actually create form. Forms are one of the tools that the master builder uses to make sure the footings are poured properly—deep enough and wide enough to withstand any assault that might occur from the outer world and secure enough to overcome any issues that might happen within as well.

Four Elements Meditation

Here is a grounding exercise. Take a moment to breathe yourself into the space where you feel completely relaxed and safe. Breathe into your heart space until you feel it is full. Now we are going to ask the each of the four elements of the planet to assist by filling us with the healing that only that element can provide. Let's use our intention to allow this to happen. First we invite the element of Air to fill us with the breath of life and all the energy that our bodies require for now and for the future and so be it. And we ask the Air element to heal our lungs and our circulatory system so that every cell of our bodies can be fully oxygenated for now and the future and so be it. Next we invite the element Fire, and ask that the Sun, the source of life fill us with its energy to burn away anything that no longer serves us, while supplying us with all the fire energy our bodies require for now and for the future and so be it. And now we invite the element of water to wash away all old emotional wounds and all unprocessed emotions and so be it. And finally, we invite the element Earth to pull us to it and hold us safely grounded for now and for the future and so be it. Now fill yourself completely with all these energies and listen to your body. Listen to the beat of your heart and notice that it speeds up as you are receiving what you require and returns to normal rhythm when you are full. And we give thanks to Mother Earth and to her elements for supporting us in every way and for supplying us with everything we require. We are forever grateful, and so it is!

Borrowed Bodies

Another definition for ground is the earth. So let's talk about why we came here. Part of our task on earth is to learn about love, and in order to do that we have to experience LACK of love. This is why we picked bodies as the tool to give us the illusion of being separate from each other, because if we remembered that we are all one, like we are at home, how could we feel any lack of love? We borrow our bodies from the earth, from the elements of the earth, carbon, water, etc. So, what are the rules when we borrow something? For example, when you borrow your friend's car, you are expected to use it, return it (with a full tank of gas) and take good care of it while you have it, right? It's the same with our bodies. How many of you ever thought about your body in that way? And when you get ready to return it to the earth when you are done with it, will you give it back in the same condition that it was when you got it, or will you give back something that is old and worn out? My guess is that few of us have taken the same care of these borrowed bodies as we would have a car borrowed from a friend. Here's another thought on that…when my mother was alive, I used to 'borrow' stuff from her all the time. Truthfully, I probably never had any intention of paying her back – I think we both knew that. How about you? And as such, perhaps we feel the same about the loans we take from Mother Earth. But, if you were to treat a loan from a bank or from the government in such a sloppy way, you would find out quickly that they were not as lenient as your mom was!

Working With Your Cells For Positive Change

Did you know that every cell has a soul? Think about it – it's a holographic universe, which means that every part of it contains the whole. As above so below, so every cell of your body contains the whole as well. This means that they all have souls. So here is a tool that connects and grounds you to your cells so that you can train them to support you in any way you'd like.

Call out to the Higher Self of the cells of your skin. Your skin is the largest organ in your body, and it replaces every cell more often than any other organ. So let's ask those cells to rejuvenate, repair and return to their Divine blueprint, erasing any wrinkles, scars or spots. Ask them to replenish collagen and elastin. Here we go:

"I now ask the souls of all of my skin cells to align with me and so be it. I ask each of you to assist me in rejuvenating and repairing the skin of my body. Please return to your Divine blueprint, remove any scars from previous wounds and any lines or wrinkles from your surface. Please replenish collagen and elastin so that your surface is smooth, firm and supple, and so be it."

Now let's talk to a different type of cell. Much research is now being done on the use of stem cells to heal the body. You can speak to your very own stem cells, just like you did with the skin. Do you have any part of your body that needs healing? Put your attention on that organ or gland. The example I will use is the thyroid gland. Many years ago I had my thyroid removed due to a diagnosis of Graves disease. I am recreating it now. Here's how:

"I now send my own stem cells to my thyroid gland and ask that they recreate it according to its Divine Perfect Blueprint and so be it."

I believe that there are particular cells that take on the role of 'team leader'. You may find it helpful to single out these team leader cells as you become more comfortable in this type of work and ask them to direct their 'team' to replicate in alignment with your desired goal.

Assemblage Point Exercise

Take three deep cleansing breaths. This exercise is going to assist you in grounding your energy into the earth, and the amazing by-product will be that you will be more centered and focused and your thoughts will become clearer. It's interesting how working with the lower chakras actually helps to clear and balance the higher ones as well.

Start by placing your attention on your navel point. Imagine a string connecting to the inside of your belly button, extending downward in the middle of your body, coming outside your body in between your legs and going into the earth beneath you. Breathe light energy into your belly button and send it down the string, causing the string to light up. Allow this light to flow into the earth. Continue to breathe into this until you feel connected to the earth with every cell of your body.

Now, locate the point in your body/field where your perception originates. It will be a ball of light that is connected to all the Light outside you. With your intention move this point to a place where you feel your power the most, again within yourself. What just happened? Did you feel your actual reality shift? Excellent! You have just reset your assemblage point to a place in your body that matches your vibration right now. As we grow in consciousness, but forget to shift our assemblage point, it's like viewing the world through glasses that are made with an old prescription. You continue to see everything from the vantage point of an old reality, rather than how it currently is for you.

Chapter Three

Who Are We Really?

Humans think that they have to know the "whole story", but we tell you that there IS no whole story because it has not yet been written. You are creating who you are with every thought, every choice you make. For too long you have allowed the beliefs and lessons of the past to limit your story, making you think you had to settle for less than what you desired. It's time to stop this insanity!

As we move forward into Unity consciousness, we remember that we are all connected to each other and to everyone and everything else. But each of us is unique and must maintain that integrity as we grow, because it is that uniqueness we carry that enables us to share the spark of the Divine that we are with the world. It is our individual sacred flame that must be protected.

In the past, we built walls of separation in order to define ourselves because we didn't know any better way. We created bodies as the ultimate separation, because they make the illusion look real. The time for walls and separateness is over, and now we are being called to find new, healthy ways to define our boundaries. Boundaries are our self-preservation and are an integral part of the Ascension process.

For as long as I can remember, I have believed that there were things outside of me that had the power to do me harm. The first and most basic (and maybe the scariest) was the belief that there was a 'devil'. I was given, or I made up, a complex set of rules and rituals to protect myself from this demon. As I grew older, my demons became more real—some of them in human form, but most lived in my own imagination. I found them in the stories I read, at Church, at school and in my own neighborhood. I was taught to be afraid. Then later when I began to study metaphysics, I learned about a whole other level of darkness—the astral where we were supposed to be very careful and make sure we didn't attract entities, and next came the ETs, who I was told could attack me and insert their dreaded implants.

Supposedly I was becoming more and more advanced, with a higher consciousness and frequency, but I was still holding on to these obsolete belief systems that made me think I was vulnerable. I was taught to surround myself with Light, to use white sage and smudge everything, and to repeat mantras to make sure I was protected from harm.

All of these beliefs were based on the fact that there was something outside myself that could harm me. I forgot who I was. The Taoist's symbol of the yin/yang is the purest representation of the truth of God. In it we can see symbolically that God contains both the dark and the light, and in the midst of the light is always a little dark while in the middle of the dark is always a little light.

We have gone past the need for artificial means of protecting ourselves. We are moving into a reality of unity, which says that we truly aren't separate from each other. But, within that unity we still have to be aware of energy—our own energy and that of everyone else. We are all both darkness and Light, and as such we can exude and receive both dark energy and Light energy. When we forget this is when we stumble. And when we aren't sure about our truth, then we can't be sure what our path is. When we lack certainty of our direction we then become vulnerable to following the energies of someone else, of taking on someone else's truth as our own. This is when we lose sight of our goal, and our ultimate goal is Ascension. When we forget where we are headed we get caught up in the material world, and there is a piece of each of us (the ego-mind, for example or the dark spot within the light of the yin/yang symbol) that wants us to fail on our quest. Forewarned is forearmed!

Compass and Square

For thousands of years, master builders have used these tools to define the boundaries of the buildings that they were creating. They are the symbols of Freemasonry, but they are your second set of Power Tools, to use as well, without any initiation or activation.

Let's talk about the compass first. What do you do with a compass? You can use it to create a perfect circle, right? This perfect circle represents the outer boundary of your personal energy field. Most of us are aware that we have other invisible bodies outside our physical bodies. Your etheric body is right outside of your physical one, an exact duplicate. Surrounding that is your emotional body, then your mental body, and finally your spiritual body on the outer perimeter. Once upon a time there was a 5th layer, the Golden Consciousness body. I have no idea what happened to it, or when, but at the time it disappeared, we were left feeling defenseless and unprotected. We began to think we had to go to great lengths to protect our energy and ourselves. Does this feel right? Does it make sense to you at some level? It is time now for you to re-activate your Golden Consciousness body. We will do this with attention and intention. So repeat after me..."I now activate my Golden Consciousness body, and so be it." And just feel the shift as this takes place.

Your other Power Tool in conjunction with the compass is the square. It will assist you in correctly delineating your TRUTH. When you can identify your personal truth—the core values that are so important to you that you would protect them at all cost— you will realize that you have actually defined your true self, without making artificial walls or separating yourself from anyone else. You have crafted your Light to be UNIQUE!

Few of us even understand what the word 'truth' means. For a long time I thought truth was finite, that once I figured it out it would be that way forever. Nothing in this life is forever.

Everything is constantly changing, including our truth. But you make a great leap forward on your path when you take the time to figure out what is important to you in the moment. My personal truth is a work in progress. Just when I think I have honed my core values into a work of art, I will find the need to expand my focus and re-write my life mission statement yet again.

What are YOUR core values? Make a list of four things that you hold to be true. If you have more than four, that's ok too, but your prime four core values form the outer walls of your personal square. They are the foundations of your authority. Remember, these are the values you live by, and they are the ideals that must be upheld in order for you to stay in integrity.

When you have identified your core values, you are ready to craft your Mission Statement. Remember in elementary school, the teacher would have you to use your spelling words in a sentence? This is how you begin to define your mission for the world. Use your core values in a sentence.

Recently, a friend of mine shared a story that is a great illustration of this point. My friend, Eric Hamel, is one of the purest Lightworkers I have had the opportunity to meet. For most of his life, he only operated from Light and love because that was all he knew. He went to a seminar where he was taught about Lemuria and the visitations to our planet by other star-beings who did things to us. He learned that we could be attacked by ETs and have implants and such done to us, and he believed what he was told. Within two days he was being attacked by ETs, implanted and tormented and fell ill. He searched for over a year to find relief, but didn't know where to turn. Finally one day he happened upon a woman who said she could stop ET torment and remove implants. He booked an appointment. When he arrived, this woman said, "You must be a powerful spirit, Eric! The King of the Reptilians came here an hour ago to ask me to tell you to leave them alone. Not just any Reptilian, but the King of all of them." My friend was amazed. He said, "No way! They are bothering me! I want them to leave me alone!" The woman then told my friend, "You believe that they are bad, but they are beings of Light just like you. Since you believe they must harm you, then they have to harm you, and they are tired of it. If you will just change your belief, then they can leave you alone. It's just that simple." He did and they did. Do you see how strong our belief systems are and how powerful our thoughts can be?

Sometimes we can be our own worst enemy. This happens regularly with respect to what we create for ourselves. Again, it boils down to belief systems, and when we believe that there is a limit to anything, we draw that line in the sand. We do it in every area of our life. We limit how much money, good health, success, joy, even love we receive, and we do it based on the core values we have set for ourselves.

Here is an example: if one of the core values you chose was financial security. When you reach the level of abundance that your subconscious mind deems to be 'financially secure', you have the potential to stop the accumulation of wealth at that point to ensure that you have reached the goal you declared. This then limits your wealth to the set-point you mentally created. And this same principle can manifest in many ways—creating loss in investment, loss of your job, etc. Designed for you, by you, to hold you in a life that is true to your values, your creation then sabotages your progress.

It is for this reason that the tools I am sharing are not meant to be used just once, then cleaned off and put neatly away. Personal growth, development and empowerment are all a process. Every time we find ourselves becoming too comfortable, we need to do a reality check to make sure that we haven't allowed that 'glass ceiling' to hold us back from having more. Likewise, when we get uncomfortable, when things appear to be going wrong, there is no room for blame, because there aren't any victims nor are there bad things that can hurt you or take your stuff. There is only YOU, so pull out the appropriate tools and make sure that your values and beliefs are in alignment with what you truly desire—not those things you don't want.

I've been playing with this concept of personal truth for quite some time. Crafting and re-crafting my core values to ensure that they really are my creations, not some plagiarized platitudes that someone else put out there. Then last night I had a very lucid dream that brought it all into perspective for me. In my dream, I was being held a prisoner in the attic of my sorority house back at FSU. In reality, there was no attic there, but regardless, there was a little door where I could go downstairs and wander around when everyone was away, helping myself to food in the kitchen, etc. At any point I could have just walked out the front door as well – but I didn't. When I began to journal this dream, I realized that it was in that sorority where I quit being ME and became what I thought I had to be in order to fit in—a pattern I have continued since 1967! As a double Pisces, I am a natural chameleon, and over the years I had molded and morphed to the point where I had lost my truth, and the values I thought were mine really weren't. We definitely teach what we need to learn!

Chapter Four

Let It Go Through Releasing

Holding on to the past holds you back from greatness. Every judgment you have made just weighs you down and turns your pathway into a steep incline rather than a gentle slope. Why would you want to make things so difficult? Certainly this was not the way it was intended, rather a game that you created. After all, the past is merely a dream. You can awaken at any point.

It's time to do spring-cleaning! We can't move into Heaven on Earth and carry with us all the baggage we have accumulated for lifetimes. In fact, why would we want to? One of the definitions of insanity is doing the same thing over and over expecting a different outcome to occur. This time, we are going to do it the right way—differently from ever before, and the outcome we will achieve is nothing less than perfection.

Since we created these bubbles of biology we call our bodies, they have become the 'closets' where we have stuffed our junk that we didn't want to deal with. "Oh, I will find a place for that tomorrow, and this is something that needs to be donated to charity," we thought. The same goes for our stories. We read a book and put it on the shelf when we are done, thinking, I might want to read this one again, it was good. "And we forget about it. Sometimes we never finish the book before we file it away." Other times we park it before we begin it, because for some reason we lose interest. Then there are the stories we read over and over. Lifetime after lifetime we just never get around to doing the work of letting go of the junk and the stories that don't serve us anymore. Playtime is over, and this stuff HAS to go!

You are all familiar with the Law of Attraction. Well, all this old residue acts like a big magnet. It attracts more of the things that vibrate at the same rate that it does – LOW. In fact, every time you tell one of your stories of wound, pain or illness, you just make more of it. It has to be that way due to the perfect consistency of the Universe. Now is the time to stop repeating those old stories, and going forward to only tell the stories of love.

The primary locations where we put the residue from pain, shame, resentment and lack of forgiveness are our chakras and our acupuncture meridians. Each of these corresponds to one of our internal organs as well, so by keeping these old wounds, we are damaging our bodies and manifesting dis-ease. You can start releasing from the outside in or the inside out. Either way, both the energetic locations and the physical ones will get clear if you are judicious in your clearing. The more peaceful way is to start with the etheric and move to the physical body, so that is what I recommend.

There are many techniques available to you for locating and clearing the past from your body, mind and spirit. There are many healers who will be willing to support you on this quest. In fact, however, we have reached a point in consciousness where when you are ready to truly claim your power as creator, you can do this by yourself. Everything can be released quickly and effortlessly without you actually having to relive or dig through the old muck in order to let it go!

All you have to do is ask! So many Masters throughout time have said this, but we were unable to hear or interpret their words. Jesus said, "Ask and ye shall receive, seek and ye shall find." This is what he was talking about. Unfortunately, until recently, our frequency of consciousness wasn't high enough for us to understand what we were being told. Listen to his words once more, and let your heart figure this out!

Now let's invite all your Angels, Teachers, Guides and the Ascended Masters to be present with you. Then ask that they present you with all your old wounds from every lifetime for liberation—easily, peacefully and harmoniously. When you feel complete with this, say the following; "I am sorry I created you, please forgive me. I love you. Thank you. I release you once and for all time." Let them go!

Another area of attachment we generally fail to examine is our attachment to belief systems. We learn and inherit these belief systems as we grow up, and many, if not all of them are no longer valid. But we were taught our beliefs by persons of authority, our parents, teachers, rulers, etc. so we believed what we were told and made these belief systems our own. Belief systems are exactly what their two-letter acronym suggests— they are B.S. As we move forward into the Ascension process, we have to let go of all B.S. along with old wounds and other junk. When we try to define anything as truth, we put it in a box, and immediately outside the box we find that there is more. There is always more, and the truth is relative. The sooner we realize this, the easier the Ascension process becomes.

Next we have to clean up our 'story'. We love to tell our story. We tell it over and over, and pretty soon we believe every word of it. But no matter how much we think we are—we are NOT our story and it has to be released. All of it. As you clear away all the parts of your own particular story, you will probably find buried under all the dust very little that is really true. Most of our stories are the compilation of the judgments of others combined with our own judgments of ourselves. You are not your story—never were, never will be. The trick is to figure out who you really are!

The Vacuum Cleaner

This brings us to our next Power Tool—the vacuum cleaner. Pick your make and model. Mine is a purple Dyson™ – a turbocharged unit that never loses its power to suck away energetic debris. It has several attachments—a crevice tool for squeezing into all the tiny places where I have hidden old B.S. and other garbage, a sweeping brush to enable me to loosen tiny particles of energy that might be stuck to my body, and a long hose to allow me to reach to the full extent of my field to find any and all old stuff that needs to go. It is really powerful. What is yours like?

Plug your vacuum cleaner into the power generator of my workshop so that you are fully connected to Source, and turn it on. Allow the frequency of love to guide it and power it to clear away everything that no longer serves you. Use all your tools to move through all your bodies, just like you move through every room of your home and vacuum away all dirt, dust, and other energy until you feel completely cleansed.

One thing I enjoy about vacuuming is watching the nap of the carpet lift and line up while I sweep it. Visualize this happening to your body and field so that you receive acknowledgement and instant gratification that you are released from the past and fully in alignment with the present moment!

Nature is nothing if not consistent. Everything in nature is ordered. It really abhors a vacuum, so the Universe will immediately try to fill any void you create with more of what was there before. Have you ever wondered why you can't just vacuum and dust your home once and be done with it? Once you release the old, obsolete stuff, you have come up with a better plan or soon you will find it all back on your doorstep again.

As you let go of the past, the beliefs that you have outgrown, all the pieces of your story etc., redo your goals and take a fresh at your core values. What is truly you and what do you need to vacuum away. Rewrite your personal mission statement. Do this exercise regularly and let it help you to guard against stagnating in your creativity. It truly is a never-ending process.

Chapter Five

Let It Go Through Detaching

One of the gifts we bring to you is the awareness of POTENTIAL. You are beginning to awaken to the portals that are opening into the quantum field, and for the first time in your history, you are able to make conscious choices from all the possibilities that exist there— not just from a single outcome that was what you thought to be the only choice. You are beginning to be able to enjoy the game of life. In fact, you are winning it.

Non-attachment is imperative as we move into higher levels of consciousness. Never before has detachment from expectation been so important. The reason for this is interesting. The field of pure potential lies in front of us in this new reality, and the options that are available are grander than we have ever been able to conceive in the past. What we can achieve is more than our wildest dreams. With our thoughts we can manifest wealth, love, and perfect healthy, beautiful bodies. With our thoughts we can create the opposite as well. Detaching is the way we will accomplish the former and not the latter.

Many things begin to go awry when we become attached to them. For example, a healer who is attached to the healing of their patient pushes the patient to the point of resistance. When this happens, the patient then shifts this resistance to the therapist, and if the therapist isn't aware of what is happening, they take it on, along with the illness or pain of the patient! Here is a higher thought for this example. If the healer could see the patient as completely free from pain or illness and hold that thought and vision until the patient can see it as well, healing could take place more easily—for both parties! As long as the healer is attached to the outcome for the patient, healing is actually blocked.

If you want to raise your vibration, you have to let go of denser attachments. This can start with the releasing of the importance of 'stuff'. What are examples of 'stuff'? Knick-knacks, jewelry, cars, alcohol, movie tickets, drama—political, religious, emotional, and the list goes on and on. It becomes a matter of choice. How important is Ascension to you? Based on your answer to this question will be what you are willing to let go of in order to achieve it. For me it is a no-brainer. After more than sixty years, I finally reached a place where I am not attached to anything anymore. Even food has lost its charge. I live in a place of trust, and I believe with certainty that all is in Divine perfection, and I'm taken care of in every way I will allow.

Another attachment is to being 'right'. This one can be more difficult to release. The rub comes from the inappropriate belief (another B.S.) that we have to help others, be a saviour. It has never been our job to help anyone else. As I've said before, you can't create in any reality except your own. But we get so attached to the things we believe to be the truth that we become blind to any other possibilities. Just look at all the religious wars that have taken place over the ages. People fought and died because they were convinced that they knew the only 'path to salvation', but the world continued turning and life went on and will continue to do so. In Tai Chi, the master averts the attack of the opponent by stepping aside. This is what detaching is all about.

The next attachment is to judgment. As humans we have become ingrained to judge. This trait just can't be carried forward into the new reality. It has to be released. Jesus said, "Judge not, lest ye be so judged." Until judgment stops, the cycle of karma will continue. This has to happen on an individual basis. Each of us has to release the need to judge anything, anyone, and ourselves. And we are definitely harder on ourselves than we are on anything or anyone outside us. As we detach from judgment we open a new door. What if everything is EXACTLY how it's supposed to be? Once this doorway is open we are then able to see more of the "big picture" and we can become the witness to the consequences of the actions of all.

We are attached to our families. We believe that our children are ours. Actually, they never were. We contracted to be the biological benefactors to bring their souls into this world, but after that, these contracts became individualized, and in some cases we didn't agree to do anything more. Our children have their own lives and their own lessons to learn. Of course, we should provide for them as best we can, but we can't dictate their path. It isn't appropriate for us to control or manipulate them either. Nor should we live our own lives vicariously through theirs. None of these is in alignment with the Universal Guidelines.

A more subtle side to the family attachment has to do with misplaced loyalty to ancestral beliefs. Have you ever noticed how certain people reach a level of income that is about what their parents had, and then can't seem to get it to go any higher? Or the man who dies at the same age that one of his parents did (think Elvis). These are just two examples of continuing a belief or action because you think you are being loyal to a parent (who am I to be more successful than my dad?)

The Reciprocating Saw (Sawzall™)

Meet your new Power Tool – the reciprocating saw. The most common brand name in the USA is the Sawzall™, made by Milwaukee Tool Company. These saws will cut through just about ANYTHING, and they are perfect for what we are doing. They are beautifully powered by the frequency of love, enabling us to sever deep connections to beliefs, people and things that we have not been able to release previously.

Detaching becomes more important when we begin to focus on conscious creation. Let's use the example of mailing a letter. You create your letter first in your mind with your thoughts.

Then you write it on paper. Next you place it in the envelope, address and stamp it. Now what do you do? You put it in the mailbox! You don't keep opening the envelope and looking at your letter, do you? You don't hold on to it and carry it around with you everywhere you go either. You DETACH from it. You must do the same with everything you desire to create. First you get clear about what you desire. Next you place your request on the cosmic. Then you detach from the thought. It rises from your mind like a beautiful balloon. Finally, you give thanks that you have received the perfect answer to your prayer. Notice, I didn't say that you give thanks for receiving the 'thing' you wanted! This is the important difference. In the new reality, we trust that we will always be given the exact response to our request.

So let's turn on our reciprocating saw, put on your protective eyewear (remember, these tools are powerful) and locate the points where you are attached to the outcome on everything you are trying to create in your life right now. Gently allow the saw to do all the work as it separates you from your attachments.

Here are some more attachments to locate and let go:

- Judgment: for the next 24 hours, stay in conscious thought and refrain from judging anything or anyone. Every time you find yourself moving into a place of judgment, pull out your saw. Listen to the sound it makes—it simply IS. Allow everything and everyone to be just as they are, and move on, content in the knowledge that it is not your job to judge anything.
- Being 'right': for the next 24 hours observe how often you feel the need to be right, to have the last word in a conversation. My mother used to say, "every time you win an argument you lose a friend". Only now do I realize how smart she was!
- Belief Systems (B.S.): Make a list of 20 things that you believe to be true. Examine each one in depth and use your

saw to detach you from every one of them. Doing this will free you to create your own belief systems

- ANY parental stuff – income, illnesses, age of death, habits
- Money
- Your Spouse or Partner
- Your home, car, furniture, toys
- Diagnosis of any illness

Chapter Six

Activating – Power Generator

The most important message for you today is that you CAN. You are more powerful than you could possibly imagine. You can change anything and everything in your reality with your thoughts. It's just a matter of replacing one thought with another of a higher vibration.

In the past, we had to be initiated in order to activate our gifts. We had to look outside ourselves to find a Master to teach us. This is an old paradigm that is being replaced by personal empowerment. You can activate all the Ascension attributes with your attention and intention. That's all—nothing more! Actually, there is a third component—NO tension. This means that you decide what you want to activate and put your attention there. You set your intention that it is so, and then you let go and let God, by putting no tension on it any further. You simply trust that what you will is accomplished for you.

Here are some of the attributes of the new consciousness that are available for activation: spiritual vision, healing, awakening of sexual bliss, infinite supply, dream travel and interpretation, true alignment, universal love, light body activation, inter-dimensional travel and communication, DNA restoration and complete acceptance. If you can conceive it, you can create it!

Sometime before written history, in fact, before compre-hended history, something happened to the genetic structure of our race. Many people, including me, believe that at some point we humans had more than two strands of DNA. My intuition tells me that there were 144 strands at one time. Nobody knows exactly why or how the "other" strands went missing, although there are plenty of scholars who will give you theories. I am going to share mine with you.

In the time of Lemuria, a continent and race of beings you might be unfamiliar with existed in the area that is now the Pacific Ocean. The inhabitants of Lemuria were a different species than the human of today. They were less dense than we are, more constructed of light than carbon-based. At some point this very advanced civilization disappeared entirely, leaving no record of its existence other than speculation (giant statues on Easter Island, for example).

I believe that these people were visited by beings of other star systems—in fact they inhabited this planet from another or other star systems, I think. For whatever reason, some arrangement was made with the visitors to modify the DNA, shutting down all but two of its strands. Perhaps these beings came to earth because they were in dire straits where they lived and they thought that mixing their DNA with ours might enable them to save their home and its inhabitants. I don't believe that there is such a thing as a 'victim', so I do believe that we must have thought that this co-mingling was in our best interest. Regardless, our species was indelibly imprinted with physical changes that took us from immortality to a much more limited lifespan, among other things.

If this sounds far-fetched to you, consider what we are doing today with genetically modifying corn, soybeans, even pigs and salmon—injecting their cells with foreign DNA using probes to create artificially mutated strains of the original. We must have agreed to this then, no different than we allow Big Pharma and Big Food to tweak our food supply to our detriment today. There had to have been a "pay-off" or we would never have allowed it.

For eons, the mass consciousness was too low to realize that there was something 'outside the box' and didn't look for more than what it already held in awareness. The Masters and Adepts knew through their initiatory, arcane teachings, so the knowledge was there, but was limited to a few 'seekers'.

Today, the consciousness of this planet has risen to the place where many new ideas are being made available to those who are looking. We are in a time of 'no more secrets'. It is amazing how when you start looking around, you will find clues everywhere. The puzzle is there for each of us to complete. It's possible that no two of us will come up with the same picture, but that's ok. Each of us will find exactly what we are supposed to find! Start your own discovery process today, if you haven't already. Accept nothing at face value, and as you begin to explore you will learn how powerful you are.

There is no loss in the Divine Plan; therefore everything that we ever had is still there, either in one of our etheric bodies or in another of our dimensional aspects. All we have to do is locate each attribute and ask that it be returned to us, along with the latent strand of DNA that is associated with it.

Put your attention on each of these attributes individually: spiritual vision, spiritual hearing, physical healing, emotional healing, awakening of sexual bliss, infinite supply, dream travel, dream interpretation, true alignment, universal love, light body activation, inter-dimensional travel, inter-dimensional communication, DNA restoral, and complete acceptance.

Ask and intend that the activation for each of these attributes take place in your reality and give thanks that it is done. I suggest that you space these activations out over a period of time so that you can enjoy the experience—perhaps do one a day or one a week. Certainly, on a daily basis, ask and intend that you receive all the energies your body requires to sustain and support it. Get creative. Look outside the box for attributes you would like to have and make them a part of your reality.

The Beings of NOW have graciously provided us with glyphs, energy drawings that can assist us in doing our own activations. They showed me 142 images that I drew and used to create the *Reconnecting Soul DNA Activation Cards*. These are available for purchase on my website, Amazon or major book retailers.

Additionally, I have created meditation movies—guided meditations using these glyphs set to the music of my friend, Jonn Serrie, Grammy-nominated composer. You will find the appropriate tool to help you.

How can all these activations and attributes apply to PHYSICAL healing is the next big question, I think. I believe that our divine human template was designed to allow us to alter every aspect of it, from the genome itself to cellular regeneration and more. When you are plugged into both the power source of the frequency of love, as well as the Divine alignments you have received just now, your physical vessel can remain in a state of harmonic accord. You achieve TRANSFIGURATION. You move from the energy of the Fibonacci spiral to the energy of the Golden Mean, and you no longer are dependent on generating power from external sources. Your body is now becoming self-sustainable. You will begin to see the effects as you become younger looking! Your hair will glow as your pineal gland emits higher frequencies! In an earlier chapter I shared several techniques for working with the souls of your cells and using your own stem cells to rejuvenate your organs and glands. How does it get any better than this!

Jesus said, "Even the least of you can do everything I do and more."

The Generator

The power tool for activating is the Generator. You are probably familiar with those emergency generators that are powered by petroleum products and generate enough electricity to get you through a power outage caused by a storm or other natural disaster. Now you have the ability to generate all the power you need to sustain yourself through any eventuality! You can activate everything you require with your intention and attention—they are your new power source.

First, let's use the generator to support your physical body.

What if you were in a state of emergency and couldn't find food or water? You could survive for days or weeks by using Universal Life Force Energy. Some call it prana, others call it different things but we are talking about energy, and all you have to do to receive it is ask. Yogis have been doing this for eons. Here's how it works: Call in your Angels, Guides, the Ascended Masters and ask them to help you. Then state, "I now fill my body with all the energy that it requires for now and for the future and so be it." Then pay attention to your body. Feel it fill. Breathe with it. When you feel full, thank all those that assisted you and close the channel and amplify with divine love. You may need to do this a lot in the beginning, but as your body becomes used to receiving what it requires in this manner, this will become second nature to you.

There are a great many benefits to living in this new reality, and one of the most outstanding is physical rejuvenation. Once you are plugged into the generator of the Divine Human Template, your cells will begin to regenerate and rejuvenate themselves quickly. As you let go of the old paradigms and B.S. that told us that we had to get old and die, you will find that you not only feel younger, but you look it too!

Chapter Seven

Accepting – Magnet

We love how you make life so difficult by refusing the gifts that come your way. You are like children at an Easter Egg Hunt. You wander around looking for the things you want, and most of the time they are in plain sight, right in front of your nose!

One of the most difficult jobs we have had to do as humans is to learn to receive, to accept without judgment. As our gifts are being activated, we have to actually accept them in order to be able to use them. This concept is quite subtle and goes back to the idea of detaching. Most of us have dreamed of what it would be like to have the powers of the Masters or the capabilities of the adepts of long ago. We believed that many of these concepts were grandiose and only existed in fairy tales, but as we move closer to our own Ascension, we find that we are actually doing many of those things. We are actually doing practical magic in our everyday lives. Sometimes we use technology, but sometimes we will do incredible things with just our minds. Until we accept our power and our divinity, nothing happens. Accepting means putting on and integrating our I AM presence; knowing that there is nothing that is beyond the capability of the human mind. When we reach this place of enlightenment, things shift.

When we don't accept something that is presented to us we block the flow of receiving, so accepting and receiving go hand-in-hand. We will discuss this more when studying the Universal Guidelines. This becomes really sticky when it comes down to receiving and accepting our spiritual gifts. Sometimes these wonderful tools can be downright daunting, even scary, and make us want to walk away from them.

This happened to me when I was a small child. Still in diapers and left alone in my crib, perhaps for a nap, I saw things that frightened me. What I didn't know then, and wouldn't have been able to comprehend anyway, was that the house I grew up in was filled with paranormal activity. The room where I slept in my little crib was right in the heart of it. I didn't find out about this until I was grown. The woman who purchased our house after my mom passed away wrote a book about her experiences there with spirits of all sorts! She said they had to close off the wing where my room had been because the paranormal activity there was so high that it was too frightening. No wonder I shut down my gifts! It took me fifty years to regain what I had filed away under a 'do not disturb' sign.

What if we were able to look at this from a different perspective? Had I been an adult, I would probably have been fascinated and done the work I do now to assist these souls to find their way to the Light. It just comes down to that old saying, "be careful what you ask for, because you just might get it!"

In order to keep the flow open, we have to graciously accept everything that comes our way, without judgment—the good, the bad, and the ugly. The proper way to do this is with a 'thank you'. When we move into the place of witnessing everything that occurs in our life rather than analyzing or judging it, accepting becomes easy, and gratitude becomes the norm.

You probably already 'get' the piece of this that relates to accepting things that are given to us, but what about things that happen to us? Because everything that occurs in our reality is a part of our creation, and therefore is a part of our learning and growth process, we must also witness and accept the actions of others as they relate to us. What I'm talking about here is accepting even the actions of others that we don't agree with. For example, if someone does physical harm to me, I don't have to agree with them that it is their right to do so, but it happened, and I must accept that it did. When I DON'T accept something that happened to me, I create a 'wound' because that incident gets stored in my makeup – in either my emotional or mental body as well as my physical one.

Let's go straight to a really heinous situation – rape. Most of the time when a rape occurs, the person who is raped actually dissociates as a coping mechanism to get through the trauma. This dissociation, while enabling survival, blocks the acceptance of what actually happened, and replaces the truth of the incident with judgment about it (did I cause this? Why me? And more.) As soon as judgment is rendered, wounding in some fashion occurs. In InnerSpeak we find all manner of energetic debris associated with thoughts and beliefs created during trauma. These wounds become blocks that at some point keep the person from having something (or everything) they desire!

Magnet

Your tool to accept is the Magnet. It gives you the ability to attract to yourself the things you desire and then hold onto them by accepting them, by becoming one with them. Have you ever noticed how non-discriminating a magnet is? As long as there is metal involved, it will hookup and accept a relationship with something else. This includes things that are physical as well as things that are not! For example, you can wipe the data off a computer disk with a magnet and you can pull the coding from a credit card or a hotel key with one as well!

You can use the magnet to wipe away the old wounds from your body, mind and spirit as easily as you can use it to accept a gift or idea you want to hold onto. Attention, Intention and No Tension is the key!

Most of us have a harder time accepting than we do giving. For the next few days, make it a point to graciously accept everything. From the smallest compliment to the largest gift, from the most joyous occurrence to the most painful, take a moment to say 'thank you'.

Chapter Eight

Listening – Digital Recorder

Humans are incredible beings. If you merely listen to another, he or she will tell you everything you need to know in the first few moments of conversation. The problem is that so few of you actually take the time to be fully present and hear what is being said. Rather you hear what you want to hear and miss the important messages.

All our answers are within us, we just have to learn to listen so that we will hear them. We ask for help all the time. Even as children we are taught to pray, "Give us this day our daily bread". And we wait and wait and wait, most of the time thinking our prayers weren't heard because we didn't get the result we expected. The disconnect happens because we were never taught how to listen for the answers!

There are two parts to prayer: asking and listening for the answer, but how few of us are able to quiet our minds long enough to allow that "still, small voice within" to be heard. We have thought for too long that in order to be answered a prayer required some sort of demonstration. Nothing could be further than the truth, although the Universe is generally very free in handing out demonstrations. Rarely does the answer come to us in the way we expect it. Perhaps that's because the Guideline of No Attachments tells us that we shouldn't be attached to how our prayer should be answered. We will never hear the answer if we don't try to listen. We will also miss the answer if we think we know how it should appear or what it should be.

For many years, there have been people who were channels. They were intuitive or psychics who tapped into other dimensions and received messages. They were not considered to be the norm, rather were looked upon as different—having 'special' gifts.

Actually, we all are channels. We can all tap into other dimensions and receive messages. We are all connected into universal consciousness or the divine mind. We are all psychic. These skills are just like our muscles. We're born with them, but we have to use them in order to strengthen them. Otherwise they waste away.

As we draw closer to the time of Ascension, it becomes more important for us to hone our intuition, our listening ability, because this will be the way of communication in the future. In the new reality, we are rapidly approaching the time when we won't even need to pay for telephones anymore! If I want to tell you something, all I will have to do is think of you and send the thought of my message in your direction. You repeat the process to reply to me. It's simple, secure and free!

Your Higher Self or soul talks to you all the time. It constantly tells you what's in your best interest and warns you about the things that aren't, but most of the time, you don't hear it. Is this because you don't know the language, you aren't listening, or you just don't care? The beautiful thing about our Higher Self is unconditional love. It never judges us for not listening, and it never stops talking. As you learn the tool of Listening, you will receive the guidance you have always wanted and you will hear the answer to every prayer.

Digital Recorder

Your tool to help you listen is the Digital Recorder. It supports you in focusing on what is being sent to you in either thought or word, so that you can be present with it and truly hear. The Digital Recorder has a noise cancelling program built into it, so it not only screens out background noise, the mind chatter that distracts you, but it also creates a permanent record of what is being recorded. This record can then stay with you until you choose to let it go. Being fully present with whoever is speaking to you is key. Acknowledgement that you have heard what is said is also very important.

Have you ever been in conversation with someone where you can tell that they are not paying attention to you? It feels frustrating, doesn't it? You don't feel acknowledged. You might even feel that you are not being taken seriously. How often have you done this yourself? When you pay attention to the speaker and acknowledge what is being said, everybody wins. Not only that, but everyone learns from the information as well as the encounter.

Let's think, for a moment, about channelling. One distraction that blocks our ability to hear messages from our soul is the judgment around it. The Judeo-Christian tradition has a lot of rules around hearing voices that can't be traced to human origins. Even though in ancient times prophets were revered, although not always 'heard', somewhere along the way, we were told that it was a sin to 'speak to the dead', and that we weren't allowed to talk to God. We bought it, hook, line and sinker, and gave our power to hear the Voice of Source away. We were even led to believe that any "voices" we might hear were evil, and that we were consorting with the devil if we listened to them. So we quit.

How can you tell whether the messages you hear in your mind are from the Light or from the dark? Your body is the barometer. How do you feel when you hear them? If it feels like love and fills you with joy, you are probably on the right track. If the message engenders fear—you probably are not. You can always ask, 'Are you from the Light?' I don't think low vibration energies can lie about their source.

Here is a tip to make yourself a better listener—count to five in your head after the speaker completes his or her train of thought. This will keep you from talking on top of him/her while allowing for any additional comments to be made. The Native Americans used a tool they called the "talking stick" to do this. If you held the stick you could talk as long as you wanted to—but only while you had the stick! It's important to remember that you can't listen and talk at the same time!

In today's world of technology, it becomes tempting to allow your Smartphone to become a distraction. When you are in a conversation with another person, in a meeting or a class—turn it OFF. There is nothing that is more important than what you are doing at the moment, and when you pay attention to the person with the talking stick, you will get the same level of respect when it is your turn!

Chapter Nine

The Level – Balancing

If you will only stay out of your own way, everything you require will be brought to you before you need it! That's the way the Universe operates, keeping balance at all times.

The Universe wants everything to be always in balance, and it strives to ensure that this is the case. Homeostasis is the property of a system that regulates its internal environment and tends to maintain a stable, constant condition. Our bodies operate in this way, as a microcosm of universal order.

There is a theory that all action follows the rule of balance as well. If you drill down deep enough, you will find that there is a counter-balance to everything that occurs. When you are able to find these energetic pairs, you have the ability to neutralize all negativity, release all fear and remove all doubt from your world. Here's how I look at the theory of balance. Any time something happens in your life, whether you perceive it to be positive or negative, the exact opposite happens at exactly the same time— somewhere. For example, someone says something to hurt your feelings. At the same moment someone somewhere is saying something good about you. All you have to do is dig deep enough and your will find that opposite occurrence. Once you acknowledge that it happened, you neutralize the charge on the hurt and release the wound. It's just that easy. The difficulty comes in remembering to dig down and find the balancing action.

Let's look at balance in a different way. Remember the axiom 'when one door closes, another one opens'? This is yet another example of balance within universal order. Florence Scovil Shinn, in her book *The Game of Life and How To Play It*, taught that there is no such thing as loss. She was striving to share her thoughts on balance. So often, though, we get caught up in our disappointment and forget to look past the surface appearance. We forget that the Universe isn't going to allow imbalance to occur, and we slip unwittingly into that place of fear, victim mentality. 'Woe is me', we lament, not realizing that a gift lies just around the corner if we will only stop whining and look for it!

There is a flip side to working with balance. When we use force instead of power, we can throw things totally OUT of balance. This happens automatically when we allow our ego-mind to drive. When we step out of surrender and think we know what is best (and usually we do this when we think we know what is best for someone else), we start trying to hammer square pegs into round holes, and they just won't fit. This out of balance energy is what limits our ability to receive all the bounty that is ours by Divine right.

The greatest example of balance exists in Yin / Yang. There is always a male as well as a female component to everything that exists. Even we humans carry both male and female energy. The left side of the body is the receptive, female side and the right is the creative, male side. Our right brain is yin and the left is yang (it's a cosmic trick – the hemispheres of the brain control the opposite side of the body!) The front of the body is yin and the back is yang. Those of us born as women work primarily with yin energy and men with yang, but we all carry both, and in order to be the best we can be, we need to be in touch with the opposite energy than our birth gender as well. Here is an interesting note: I don't believe that our brains were always divided. It's my thought that at some point in the evolution of the human, we carried both energies in complete balance, and our brains functioned without the cleft, with all parts communicating at all times. When did the change occur that broke down communication and left us believing that we had to have something outside ourselves in order to be successful? Certainly before present history and Homo sapiens. But there are no victims. I believe we agreed to this evolutionary change in order to master some lesson.

We experience discomfort when we are out of balance in our human vessels. And we must intend that we find that balance if we want to avoid involving our physicality. The balance is between the obvious, the male and female aspects of ourselves, but there is a third component – that of the child. When our Inner Child is out of balance with its male/female aspects, it is no different than a little human child who is out of control. That scared Inner Child is the one who is causing the upset in our outer world as we move higher and higher in consciousness. Little children don't like change. They want stability, and when they feel ungrounded, they 'act out'!

My Inner Child has been trying to get my attention for months to show me the areas where I was out of balance – pain, illness, and I wasn't listening! So it began to throw tantrums. How do you deal with a four-year-old who is having a tantrum? Today's kids respond best to love and consistency. Tell your child that you are in charge as its parents – both mother and father, actually. Tell it that you will protect it at all cost as you move together upward and into a much better space. Tell it that it is loved beyond all comprehension – and FEEL that for yourself!

Exercise – Brain Balance

Here is a meditation you can use to balance the hemispheres of your brain, to grow new neural synapses and facilitate faster communication between the right and left-brains:

> Prepare yourself by relaxing into a meditative state. Use your breathing or whatever relaxation technique you prefer as you become fully present in your body. Allow all tension to drain out through the soles of your feet. Scan yourself to find any

places where you are storing any pain, dark energy or stuck feelings and release these now. Put your attention on the pineal gland in the middle of your head, and with your intent, stimulate it to release the hormonal secretion MANNA. Allow these secretions to flow into every area of your brain. Let them wash over every surface, into every fold and crevice. Now ask your brain to return to its Divine Blueprint. Ask it to heal the separation of the hemispheres and reconnect all neural networks from both halves. So Be It! Now rest while your brain obeys your decree. Feel the energy as it moves back and forth inside your head. Enjoy the excitation as the New is brought into you. Remember, remember. In your DNA the memories are stored of life before 'the split'. You can remember how powerful you were when you were completely balanced, and you can bring those feeling memories forward into the Now. This is the present moment—this is the NOW.

Chapter 10

The Copier – Sharing

Each of you has SO much to share with the world. You are beginning to wake up from the nightmare of "lack" and fear. Fantastic things await each of you who realizes that giving and receiving go hand in hand—one is not better than the other.

The theme for the new reality as we move forward is collaboration. That's the foundation of Unity Consciousness. Now we will truly understand the meaning of cooperation. For the last 26,000 years as we lived in duality, we feared that there wasn't enough to go around, but that fear has only served to become a self-fulfilling illusion. We bought into belief systems of lack and struggle. The time for this is coming to a close. We are returning to a simpler paradigm. Remember how the pilgrims shared their bounty with the Native Americans on the first Thanksgiving? This is an example for each of us as we step into these higher frequencies. The global financial structures are changing. The Mayans and Hopi predicted this many years ago. If we want to live in abundance, we must be willing to share what we have with others and learn to do business in new ways. In the 19th century, when we were primarily an agrarian society, we shared what we had with our neighbors. If my farm produced an overabundance of eggs, I would share them with you in exchange for grain, and so forth. Nobody went hungry, nobody hoarded and life was peaceful. In the southern United States, it became traditional to bring some of that bounty to church on Sunday to share with others at what was called "dinner on the ground". Times of joy and sadness were occasions for bringing food to share with friends and neighbors. Unfortunately, many of these traditions have been neglected or forgotten, and it's time to resurrect them. The Universal Guideline of Giving and Receiving states that when we give freely, we receive freely. If we share with others, we, too, will benefit. We stand alone no longer! Each of us has at least one unique gift to share with the world. It's our job to share our gift by living every day in our truth. How difficult could that be? In times past, it was extremely difficult, because the frequency of mass consciousness wasn't high enough to support us. Times have changed, and every day, our vibration—as well as that of the Earth—increases. Once you realize this, and open to possibilities, it becomes more difficult NOT to share your gift. I find that when I step away from integrity in any area, I am quickly (sometimes rudely) reminded that this isn't in my highest interest, and I actually see the appropriate thought or action so that I can change my course.

Once you've gotten what you asked for, it is time to share the fruits from your bounty. The ten percent rule is a good one. Take some off the top of whatever the universe provides for you and share it with someone else. It doesn't have to be money all the time. If you asked for love, then give love to someone who could use it. If you asked for a job, create some work for someone who's down on their luck—or keep your ears to the rail and pay attention for other jobs which might match up to someone you know who is looking for work.

Another thought about sharing—pay forward to those who feed you spiritually! If someone inspires you, support their work. If you find a book which lifts you, buy another copy and give it to a friend. It doesn't have to be money—everyone loves a gift, even if it's just a sweet note of gratitude. No good deed ever goes unrewarded. That's how the Universe works!

The Copier
The power tool to assist you in sharing is the Copier. You can make as many copies of your blessings and bounty as you want – the paper is unlimited…you can print money now, if you desire

with this fantastic machine that is plugged directly into Source. You can also copy much more with this very flexible tool. You can copy your ideas, love, beauty, your strengths and abilities. The more copies you make, the more you have for yourself as well. Isn't this FUN?

Here is how it works:

When you help someone else, that energy flows back to you and makes more of the same. This energetic exchange creates more of the same in all areas of your life, and more important—there is no order of magnitude in sharing—a smile generates as much energy as a gift of money!

Sharing Exercise

Try this for the next day or two:

Ask each person you come into contact with to share with you one of their aspects that you admire and would like to duplicate within yourself. For example, if your boss demonstrates great organization skills and the ability to look outside the box for solutions to problems, tell her and ask her to share that ability with you. If your friend is very compassionate, ask him to help you to be more like him. If your spouse is able to focus extremely well and always completes tasks, you might like to be able to do so as well. You will be amazed at the results!

Chapter Eleven

The Dream of Conscious Creation

There isn't anything that you can't have, if you just set your mind to it. You merely seem to have forgotten how simple the steps to manifesting are. We are happy to remind you, now that you ask!

During a recent meditation I asked to be taught the steps to instant manifestation. This is something I have been working on for several years—since the release of my book, *Reframe Your World*. I am very good at manifesting actually. I have everything I require and more; living in heaven on earth, happy, healthy and self-sufficient. But, I don't actually know how I manifest. I have read all the books; understand the Universal Laws—even lecture on them, done every technique, but the results still tend to be haphazard and unpredictable. If the Laws are the laws, the results should be very predictable and consistent, but mine aren't, so I must be missing at least one of the steps. The meditation turned into a nap, but I received a huge amount of information as a dream while I rested.

Here is what I learned that day. The first step of conscious creation is to give up all attachment to the results of what I want to manifest and the timeframe I expect to see them. In fact, every belief about whatever I am looking to receive must be erased completely. The object of my intention must be a blank slate. Mike Dooley said it perfectly when I opened my daily 'Message from the Universe' one morning, "Ever notice how when someone dreams of happiness, abundance, health, romance, or friendship, they never have to wonder if it's in their best interest? But when someone dreams of a specific house, employer, love interest, deadline, dollar amount, or diet fad, they often end up contradicting themselves." (For more of these wonderful messages, visit www.TUT.com and register.) Keep your end results general. Everything else is just a how. What I am learning is that "how" is not my job! Sometimes the way my manifestations demonstrate themselves is nothing short of amazing, and more outrageous than I could ever have conceived.

Generally we humans don't realize how attached we are to an outcome. We even think we are being open and general as we request a new car, new job, new lover, etc. For decades, books and teachings on manifesting have told us to be very specific about our desires, and I have ascribed to those teachings over time, just like most of us. And my results have been inconsistent. It would be interesting to go back and document whether many of the things I've 'consciously created' were things I was general about or ones where I got extremely explicit. Therefore, we have to stay very conscious while we are working this magic of manifesting.

Step two is to trust that I can have exactly what I require to meet my needs and whatever the end result is—it will be perfect, even though it might not look like what I expected when I started the process. This is a huge leap of faith; complete surrender. We are so used to having to take care of ourselves, setting goals, being explicit, etc., that this is extremely hard for humans to do.

Our mortal mind is sure that it knows what is best for us, and we tend to defend those goals and objectives to death (literally!) Giving over the reins to something seemingly outside ourselves feels like insanity the first time we do it. But surrender places us in alignment with our Higher Self, which absolutely is part of us. When did we start to believe it wasn't? Why would we give away our power? What made us think we didn't deserve to have what we wanted? We seem to be stuck in the fear that in order to able to do that, we will have something taken away that we think we need. This leads to what I call crisis mode, causing our adrenals to kick in and our connection to our power center to shut down. Totally counterproductive! It's actually a syndrome that makes us believe that any change will probably cause loss, so we become rigid and afraid of change and then we get STUCK.

Once the intent is expressed to the Universal Mind, things are being set in motion and manifesting is starting to happen. This brings us to step three—throw emotion into the mix. This is like adding fuel to the fire. Our emotions are a form of energy, so they are fuel. When the manifestation object is something we are passionate about, the emotion flows easily. If we don't believe it's truly possible for us to create whatever this is, however, fear becomes the dominant emotion, and we move into a place of lack.

Consider the Old Testament story of the Israelites wandering in the desert for 40 years. They ran out of food and were starving, so to say that they were passionate about asking their God to provide food for them is an understatement. The emotion they put out was desperation, and it worked just fine, and they were fed. Many times we are also led to create from desperation, but if we would have consistency in our results, our goal should be preparation. In this manner we can stay focused on our direction and work with the Universe to ensure that we have what we require before we reach a place of crisis. Manna is a gift. The first manna was a gift to a starving band of wanderers. It satisfied their hunger. Today manna has the ability to do the same—to satisfy your hunger to create. Jesus said, "I can give a man a fish and he will be hungry again tomorrow. I can teach him how to fish and he will never hunger again."

This requires diligence and commitment on our part. The commitment is to staying in the present moment and within the Circle of Surrender as opposed to the Triangle of Fear and Control (for more information, see my book, *Reframe Your World*). Try using Joy as your constant emotion! Joy is the perfect platform for creating the reality you desire. The law of attraction says that what you put out to the Universe is what you will receive in return, so if you live in joy, you emit the frequency of joy, and everything you attract will also carry that same frequency. Another aspect of manifestation that needs to be understood is what is the frequency or vibration of creation. The frequency of creation is love. In order to hasten the attraction of the object of your desire to you, it's a good idea to match the frequency of creation with your own. How can you accomplish this? By asking! Ask the Universe to fill you with the vibration of love and then open your heart to receive it. Feel it flow into the core of your being and keep asking until you can hold no more. It's the Law of Attraction at work!

Next, don't allow anything to pull you from your intended direction. Once you set your intent and add your emotion, you are well on your way to success. This is the hardest part of the process—not succumbing to fear. It's so easy to slip out of joy and into worry. The distractions are everywhere. It would be a lie to say that staying in joy is simple. At any point, your shadow is there to remind you to be aware of it, and this is the place in the manifesting process where it is most important to stay upbeat so that positive energy keeps flowing into your creation so that you receive it in the physical quickly. Think about baking a cake. What would happen if you carefully mixed all the ingredients placed them in the pan and into your pre-heated oven, then turned the oven off? You'd get a flat result, gooey in the middle and not at all what you wanted! Your state of joy is what keeps the oven at the right temperature to allow your manifestation to bake to perfection.

The example I was shown in my meditation was relative to food. I was given Manna. It looked like a loaf of bread, beautifully prepared and perfectly baked. When I broke the loaf and took a piece to eat, it melted in my mouth, just like cotton candy, and it provided me with all the nutrition and energy my body required. I was told that I would receive enough for my daily needs, as well as the needs of my family and pets, but I wasn't to share it outside of my immediate family. Manna is an individual gift, and we each have to figure out how to create it to meet our own specific needs. I was told it wasn't a commodity to be sold, but I could teach others the process of making it.

The final step in the creation process is to actually become what you wish to create. In the story, the Israelites ate the manna. They became it because they consumed it. You know the law of attraction – so you must consume and become the vibration of what you desire. If you want love, become love. If you want money, become money.

Manna is synonymous with whatever is manifested as a conscious creation, and the possibilities are unlimited. Think about the ramifications of just creating manna to feed oneself: no longer is money required to purchase food, so that piece of one's disposable income is freed up for other uses. No time would need to be expended to figure out what to eat that day, or find the ingredients or prepared food, or cook, or even to eat. Therefore, large chunks of time are freed up as well as money! But there is more, and this is where most people go into fear. If people aren't purchasing food, the supply chain is disrupted, along with financial markets, etc. Once this gets figured out and large numbers of people realize that they can manifest every-thing they both desire and require, our global economy will change radically. Nostradamus, the Mayan Elders, and many others have predicted this for thousands of years. Until recently, I thought this meant disaster, but now I am figuring out that what these Masters were telling us is that there is a better way, one of collaboration and unity, and this will erase lack from reality.

The major obstacle here is figuring out what we really want! Because the way the Universe presents our manna to us isn't necessarily how we might have imagined it. God's answer to every question is always yes. We just have to listen... We are living in a time of tremendous change. Never before in recorded history has there been so much turmoil on a global level. The proportion of this is in part due to the immense population of the planet, as well as to media coverage, which allows every little ripple to be felt by more people than ever before. Most of us are resistant to change because we have old programs and beliefs that tell us that change will be hard or painful. It is a human characteristic to resist change. Our ego selves operate at the level of a four or five-year-old child—one who wants everything to always remain just as it is. But, the "same old, same old" doesn't serve us in the new reality, the consciousness of unity. Things have to change. Just like the snake that sheds its skin when it becomes too snug to allow for growth, we must transform so that we can grow as well, both personally and as society.

We are being tested on the lesson of personal empowerment— a cosmic "pop quiz", if you will. If you are reading this book, you have been on a path of raising your own consciousness and moving toward finding your purpose. Probably you have been using the Law of Attraction to create what you want in your life. Then WHAM, the rug is pulled out from beneath your feet! Global financial markets tumble and enter crisis mode. Jobs are lost. Disaster strikes in the Gulf of Mexico. Homes and the perception of security are in jeopardy for many. Fear and unrest abound. Sometimes the test appears as illness or pain. You might be asking yourself, 'How did I go wrong?'

Fear is an illusion of our ego. The ego-self is that part of us that is aware of material concerns and physical wellbeing. Your soul, however, knows and understands that this is all part of Divine Plan. Now is the time for us to resolve this dichotomy. All existing structures based on duality must change and old paradigms of greed or lack have to fall away at this point to create space for a new reality of love, oneness and 'plenty'. We have known about this shift for a long time. Many have prayed for it, and now we sit in the hours before the dawning of the New Age. Trust me when I tell you that you ante'd up all your chips to be here now so that you could experience this, so be not afraid!

The easiest way to move through these turbulent times is to stay centered and grounded in your personal faith—trusting that the Architect of this grand plan holds true to The Word. You are safe, and you will be provided for in every way. As you release all your old beliefs that are out of alignment with the new reality—thoughts of fear, lack, pain, and disease—you prepare the way to create the truth for yourself. You must be judicious, now more than ever before, to monitor your thoughts constantly to remove any negative ones before they are allowed to surface. If you become aware of one that might manifest an outcome you wouldn't desire, re-language it immediately. For example, change 'I'm not healthy' to 'In the past I wasn't healthy, but now I am healed.' In this way you project a positive outcome and state your truth. Remember—it's all about choice. You can choose in every moment whether to be positive or not, and what you choose will absolutely shape your reality.

Examine everything that crops up in your life and doesn't feel like love, peace or joy. Your body is one of the greatest barometers you own. If you tune in, it will tell you exactly where you are at any moment, so check in with your feelings constantly. When you find something that just doesn't 'feel' good, find the lesson and the blessing in whatever it is, because there always will be both. If you don't find the lesson—it will come around again with higher stakes. Learn it when it is presented as a carrot and don't wait for the stick!

There has never been a more perfect time for you to read this book! Use it as your stabilizer. Anchor into the tenets you will find here to keep you focused on the positive. Every moment of every day is a choice. As it says in *A Course In Miracles*, 'I can choose PEACE...'

Hologram of Creation

Close your eyes for a moment. Take a long, deep breath—in through your nose and out through your mouth. Just let go and trust. Allow your imagination to expand. Create a giant clear ball in front of your field of vision—GIANT. Start placing the things you desire inside this ball. Notice that it looks like a snow globe, right? You can fill it up with silver trays of money, new cars, new houses, your perfect job, a vacation to the Caribbean, whatever you want. Be creative! When you think you have everything in there that you could possibly ever use, add three more things.

Now, watch as your ball of possibilities begins to rise into the air. As it lifts it gets larger and larger and floats higher and higher. Give it to God and say, "These things and more are mine now. Thank you! They come to me now, under Grace in a perfect way and I am blessed." Let it go. You don't need to repeat this process again, because it is done. (...and you ARE blessed!)

What is your dream?

There isn't anything that is outside the realm of possibility for you to create in your life. All you have to do is decide where you want to begin. You remove distraction from the equation if you focus on a single manifestation project at a time. This is no different from the way you program your GPS to get you to your destination on a trip. First you decide where you want to go. With our manifestation project, however, you are looking at an end product of reality, not necessarily a destination. For example, if the areas of your life where you are looking to make enhancements are career, weight, health, finances and relationships, choose one as your focal point. You are not limited in the things you can create; so now is the time to make your complete wish list, and then prioritize. Think BIG! Get outside your usual comfort zone. Stretch your imagination. The only limits are the ones you place on yourself.

We are in such a phenomenal period for creating. The consciousness of the planet is higher than it has ever been before, and the results of your thoughts are coming in so quickly it's almost hard to fathom. This morning when I was cooking breakfast, as I chopped veggies for our omelette, I realized that all the garlic had spoiled. I thought to myself, when we go into town this morning we must remember to buy garlic. An hour later, we were off on our run to do errands and passed a farmer's market at the county courthouse. It looked appealing so I pulled in. The first booth I came to was selling only—guess what— garlic! Beautiful purple garlic from the farmer's organic garden, and it was so much better than what I would have found at the grocery.

I have found that my best results occur when I take this process very lightly. Once I said, "I miss going places on airplanes." Within two months I had manifested a new job making a great salary and flying once or twice a week to appointments in a fourteen state territory. It is as though the Universe is best able to create for us when we allow a large palette for It to paint on. This is a perfect example of not having an attachment to an outcome. In fact, I didn't even realize I was creating a manifestation. I merely thought I was making conversation with a friend! So, this is a BIG clue for you as you start this process. Pick an object to pull into your awareness that has a vague outline so that something larger than your mortal mind can color in between the lines for you.

Imagine yourself relaxing in a swimming pool containing hundreds of pool toys. Which one would you want to play with? What float would best support you as you sun yourself? How about a Pina Colada to refresh yourself? This is what the universe of potential resembles! All you have to do is swim over and grab your toy, climb onto a colorful raft and hold out your hand so the cabana person can provide you with a drink!

Awareness is the point where manifesting begins—not with the awareness of what you want, but rather with the awareness of where you are in the moment, what you have right now. Once you have the awareness that you are complete in the now, you are ready to step into the process of manifestation. If you plan to do your creating for something in the future, that is where it will stay—in the future.

Let's start with now. What is the most important thing to you right this minute? It can be anything—there is no judgment. Is your focus on money? Health? Relationships? Career? Where you put your attention is what you will create in life.

In order to get to the crux of what is important for you, begin by listening—listening to your own inner voice. In fact, nothing can be accomplished until you do. This is a huge step, and many of us find that we not only don't know how to do it, but as we focus on this, we are surprised to learn that we don't have a clue what listening means. We hold all the answers inside, and they are readily accessible if we know where to look (or listen, more precisely). Generally, however, we have a hard time figuring out what we want to have first. You can use your feelings to help you get a handle on what is the most important. A good guideline is excitement. When you think of something do you get fired up and feel good, or are you merely neutral? Does a smile appear on your face? Do you sit up a little straighter in your chair?

Here is a tool to assist you in figuring out what is your priority. In the following grid, number these items in the order of how much they EXCITE you, from 1 - 12. Really get in touch with your feelings before you begin. This exercise allows you to see where your awareness is based on how much emotion you generate relative to the particular topic. We are going to examine the role of emotion in manifestation in another chapter, but first we have to choose the singular item to create in the now. There is no right or wrong as you order these items.

- Money
- Friends
- Love
- Career/job
- Spirituality

- Home
- Exercise
- Diet/nutrition
- Health
- Hobbies
- Play
- Rest.

Going forward, we will work with your top three areas where you would like to create a shift. Take a minute to congratulate yourself. What you have just done is HUGE! So much energy is wasted when you don't have focus. When you are attempting to create change in too many areas of your life at the same time, the cosmic support that flows as a response to your prayers can feel overwhelming. It manifests as chaos, actually. This fun, little tool just helped you sharpen your focus and use the Universal flow to your advantage.

Here is another important piece to the puzzle: now that you have prioritized the areas where you desire change, check in with your Higher Self. Change is always easier and faster if what you want to create is in alignment with your life purpose and your highest good, rather than just a desire of your ego. Ask your Higher Self if your desire is in your best interest as well as in line with the highest direction for your life. Then LISTEN... Really get quiet and feel the answer in your heart. If what you get is a "no", rethink what your needs are! You will find that your tools in this creation game are intention and attention. Therefore you will put your attention on the areas you select that are in agreement with your Higher Self, and then you will set your intention to receive what you desire from the Universe, and so be it!

Have you ever looked at your digital clock and seen repetitive numbers such as 3:33, 4:44 or 11:11? Did you wonder if there was anything special about this? I consider these displays of Master

Numbers to be 'cosmic winks', little taps on the shoulder to bring us into the present moment and offer the opportunity to do some conscious creation. You can use them as signals to remind you to do your homework and create something wonderful for yourself on one of the target areas you have just selected, or just be thankful for the blessings you have already received. Gratitude is like the cement that holds the manifesting process together, so the more you express how grateful you are, the more the Cosmic smiles on you with bounty and blessings! Keep your eyes peeled for the hints that surround you!

In numerology, each number has an energy associated with it, and when numbers are grouped together that frequency is amplified. Throw your own desires into this mix and you have a perfect palette for manifesting miracles. Please note that these are my ideas about the frequencies of numbers, and are certainly not based on science. (You may smile here!)

Here are some ideas to play with when numbers begin to appear in your reality, and if you set the intent to have this happen, I assure you that it will:

- The number 2 vibrates to relationships, so when you see 2:22 on your clock, put your attention on what you desire in the area of relationships—either finding a new one or making your existing one stronger.
- The number 3 holds the frequency of communication, so when you see 3:33 it is a signal to focus on self-expression and sensitivity.
- The number 4 is what I call the Master Builder number, so at 4:44 look at what you are trying to create and focus on that. Think of yourself as the architect of your life and allow your imagination to blossom into a grand plan. This is not the time to think small. 4:44 is telling you that you have huge potential ready to unfold. 444 is also considered to be the number of the Angels, so when you see this

combination, just know that you are surrounded with celestial love.

- Five is the number of freedom, so at 5:55 you can examine the areas of your life where you desire to have more freedom.
- I left the number one for last, because you have two opportunities to create "one" things, at 1:11 and 11:11. These are the most powerful of the master numbers. They represent unity and personal growth. Eleven is the Master Number that reflects the transformation of the physical into the Divine. Pay attention when you see either set, because the Universe is telling you that you are in the process of raising your consciousness. If you listen closely, you might just hear that "still, small voice" whispering the secrets of the ages in your ear!

After you have found clarity on what you desire in the appropriate area, surrender it to Spirit and just let it go. Allow the Universe to figure out what's best for you in response to your request and present it. I always add, "This, or something better, comes to me now in a perfect way, thank you!" Remember, the 'how' is not your job! All you have to do is decide upon the 'what' and leave the rest up to the Divine. Remember, surrendering means letting go. This is the point in the process where you are called to relinquish control and trust that everything you desire has already begun its journey into manifestation.

Think back to the example we looked at earlier about what happens when you decide to mail a letter? You put it in the mailbox and forget about it. Manifesting is the same – it's like mailing your request to the Cosmic and trusting that it will be delivered on time. Certainty will replace doubt if you are able to let go of your attachment to a specific outcome. There is a force much greater than you that can take over when you release control, and it creates solutions that you would not have considered on your own.

Once you release your creation to the Universe, take a minute to give thanks that you have already received it along with a multitude of other blessings. Notice how light this makes you feel. You have pulled yourself fully into the present moment when you stop to be grateful, and the present moment is all there is. It is the place where you stand in your power and can create the reality you desire and deserve, and nothing can stand in your way.

In summary, then, you have to a) listen, b) ask and then c) receive. It's that simple!

Let's step back now to awareness. Remember that I said that where your awareness is, that is what you will create? So, let's take health for example. Perhaps you have been ill and are looking to heal your body. So you move through the process we've talked about and you have released your desires to the Universe. If you continue to put your attention on the aches and pains, though, you will keep them in your reality and you will block your own manifestation process! You have to let the past go at the point when you release your desires for manifestation. This isn't the easiest thing for us to do, is it? I chose pain as the example here because it's really easy for pain to get our attention and hold it! But in this new paradigm of manifestation, we have to stay vigilant if we are to receive our creations quickly. Do what you need to do (healthy things only) to take your focus off the things that you don't want, such as pain. Distract yourself. You will find that this is easier than you think. It's all about staying in the present moment, because in the present, there is no pain, no fear, no lack.

Let's look at how this works in other areas, such as wealth and love. You have to release your focus on what you don't have. This includes talking about it! The more you bemoan your loneliness or how you don't have enough money to pay your bills, guess what happens? You stay lonely and short of cash. They become your story that doesn't serve you. Remember what I said about God's answer to every questions is always yes? We are so used to talking about our problems. It's almost as though we thought that the more we discussed them with the most people that maybe we were spreading them thinner and they might actually disappear. Wrong! The more we talk about what we don't like about our lives, the longer we stay stuck in that place.

Another piece of awareness around talking involves refraining from telling others about the things you are looking to create. Keep your manifestations to yourself until they appear in your life. Don't tell anyone what you are doing—not your spouse, your best friend or your co-worker. It's tempting to do so, because you are excited. You have unleashed a lot of energy, but one of the most sabotaging things you can do in this process is to talk about it.

Why is this, you are thinking? Everyone you tell your dream to will have their own thoughts about it—some positive, some not so positive. Their energy will attach to your dream and lower its vibration. This might actually cause you to doubt your own ability to receive and shift you away from that certainty that fuels the creation process. It's difficult to keep our dreams to ourselves. We get excited about the things that fuel our passion. The catch is—keep the passion flowing and allow the manifestation to occur. There will be plenty of time for sharing your success with others then!

When your manifestation appears is the appropriate time to tell the world. Shout the news of your demonstration from the rooftops! The Universe loves it when you are so grateful that you share your news with others. This is, in fact, a form of gratitude. Remember, choice is one of our most precious gifts, and in every moment we can choose to have life and have it more abundantly.

- Starting today, keep your conversations focused only on the positive. Consciously monitor every word that comes out of your mouth and every thought in your head. This one is difficult, because many of us have allowed complaining to become a habit, but it isn't impossible if you really want to make a shift in your life!

- Don't allow yourself to get sucked into another person's misery either! Remember the 'lowest common denominator' rule? Other people will pull you down to their level and before you know it you will be talking about your own miseries, defeating your purpose.

- Learn to say 'no' to negativity. If a co-worker or friend wants to discuss their drama, disconnect. Find an excuse to move away. 'Oh my gosh, I'm running out of battery on my cell phone – gotta go!' You are freeing your friend and you are freeing yourself.

- Give yourself the gift of YES! Forget about the past and all the times you felt like you got the short stick. When you step into conscious creation you receive an unlimited supply of 'do-overs. If you don't like what happened a moment ago (or yesterday) change the thought that made it so, re-think and make it be like you truly want it to be! Keep doing this until the results look like what you desire.

Chapter Twelve

You Aren't The Only God!

Humans are more afraid of their own power than any other species in the Universes. Once you release the old beliefs that have engendered this level of fear, you will realize that you hold within your very DNA the ability to transform your entire reality, to manifest abundance and to live in complete peace.

The power is yours as Creator to bring into existence the exact reality you dream of. Once you remember that you are god, you can harness that power and make things happen. But you can only create in your own reality, and it is important that you remember that you are not the ONLY god. Every one of us on this planet is god – made in the image of God. We can only create in our own reality, and not the reality of anyone else. This is one of the things we tend most to forget.

We want something to happen that involves someone else, then we become disappointed when whatever it is doesn't come about. Why is this? The desires of all concerned must be in alignment in order for anything to be created. Generally we aren't aware of all the components of the equation that is involved in creating what we want. Additionally, everything must happen according to the time plan of all concerned, and it must also be for the highest good of all involved. It's like what happens when dominos are standing in a line and the first one is tipped and they all fall over. It can be frustrating to try to manifest when these principles aren't figured into your plan.

Here is an example: you desire to attract your Beloved. You have done a lot of inner work to clear away your debris and learn to love yourself. You have prepared a place in your life for this person. But time passes and he or she doesn't show up. What's wrong? Nothing—absolutely nothing! As soon as you are ready for your Beloved, the Universe presents him or her, but what if that person is married, involved or otherwise committed? If he or she is the 'one', those interfering obstacles have to be neutralized for the highest good of all involved. Sometimes this takes time... If you are like me, you probably get really impatient waiting for the wheels of creation to turn. When creation doesn't involve another or others, you may find that your manifestations might even appear to be instantaneous!

Learning About Love

You came here to this planet to learn about love. Where you existed before this there was only love. God was all there was, and all souls were part of that. It was all energy. The only way you could learn about love was to experience the lack of it. At Home, because God was the creator, He/She took care of all the souls and filled them with love. Therefore it was impossible to feel the lack of love. Here we arrived and 'borrowed' these bodies so that we could see what it would be like to be separate from that love (and everyone and everything else). Now we are trying to remember why we did this. What could we possibly have been thinking! Along with these bodies came the erasing of all the memories of Home. We even left behind our 'playbook' so that we couldn't remember the rules of the game of life.

There are paradigms that govern how the universe operates. They are constantly at work, whether we are aware of them or not. For most of recorded history, these paradigms were considered to be laws, the Universal Laws. The interesting problem is that these 'laws' aren't the ones we are taught in school (or even Sunday school,) so most of the time we don't understand how they are impacting our daily life. We just think stuff happens by coincidence, but there really are no coincidences. We are now moving into such a new level of reality, that going forward we should look at these laws as guidelines, because if we are unaware of them or choose not to follow them, we will be locked into lower vibrations and our manifestations will be blocked or slowed. Therefore for the purpose of this book, and going forward, I will be calling these 'laws' the Universal Guidelines.

Three of these major guidelines are Attraction, Synthesis and Economy of Force. These play together in the world of manifestation. They are the process by which manifestation takes place, and they work either against us or in our favor, depending on how we use them. We will tackle each of them individually now.

The Guideline of Synthesis

The aspect of will is a difficult concept to understand. It demonstrates the fact that all things - abstract and concrete - exist as one. This paradigm operates from the position that each thought is a unit of God's thought, and as such is connected to everything and everyone else in the Universal Mind, and not the differentiated process that we have always thought our own evolving system to be. We are a part of this guideline as well. This is a holographic Universe, and as such, each of us exists as a part of the whole. Synthesis is the sum total, the center and the periphery, and the circle of manifestation regarded as a unit. It is your will in alignment with the Universe, and only when your will is in alignment with the good of the whole can you consciously create what you want. This is the point of realization of I AM, and once it is accepted and understood, it becomes the primary guideline of a conscious Man/Woman. We are all part of the whole. Everything we do affects everyone and everything else. When you assist another to win, you win as well. In fact, everything you do should be win-win. In this new reality, synthesis leads to and supports collaboration.

The Guideline of Economy of Force

This paradigm is the Activity aspect of manifestation. This is the energy that adjusts all that concerns the material and spiritual evolution of the cosmos to the best possible advantage and with the least expenditure of force. It rules the physical atom, and makes perfect each atom of time and each eternal period and carries all onward and upward and through, with the least possible effort with the proper adjustment of equilibrium and with the necessary rate of rhythm. It is the metaphor of 'if it's easy for me, its right for me' — my personal mantra. Unevenness of rhythm is really an illusion of time and does not exist in the cosmic center. We need to ponder this, for it holds the secret of peace, and we need to grasp the significance of that word, for it describes the next racial expansion of consciousness, and has a hidden meaning. The person who aims at providing a point of contact between conditions of chaos and ones that work for constructive ends and order, should likewise use that most necessary factor of common-sense in all that s/he does. This involves always obedience to this guideline of economy of force. Where it is present, time will be economized, energy will be wisely distributed, excessive zeal will be eliminated, allowing the Universe to depend upon an aspirant's sagacity and thus find a helper. We don't have to do it alone anymore. Truthfully, we never did!

This guideline implies that being and doing need to be in balance. Being is feminine and doing is masculine, and when the two are balanced, equilibrium is established.

The Guideline of Attraction

This is the basic governing influence of all manifestation, the Love aspect, and it governs the Soul aspect as well. Fundamentally, this guideline describes the compelling force of attraction that holds our solar system in its place. It holds our planets revolving around our central unit, the sun. It holds the lesser systems of atomic and molecular matter circulating around a center in the planet, and that of the subtle bodies coordinated around their microcosmic center.

Where you put your attention and what you believe is what you will create. For example, when the salesperson puts their attention on manifesting sales, or appointments, etc. these things begin to flow to them, and the more passionate the rep is about doing their job, the more they are open to receive. This is why it is important to plan the week, plan the day and then work your plan. The more appointments a rep sets and does, the more appointments they will get going forward. The more sales you win, the more sales you WILL win. Success breeds success.

Another large implication of this guideline is that you can only create what you already are energetically! Therefore, if you desire to manifest anything, you must first hold the energy of that inside yourself. As soon as you do that, you will create it in your world. Using I AM statements will assist you in this process. For example, I AM Self-Love is one of the most important ones you can use. When you truly love yourself, the Universe responds with love, with energy that fuels the creation of all your desires.

Other Guidelines

There are many other Universal guidelines that will come into play as we delve more deeply into the principle of active manifestation. Each of them works with a different aspect of reality, and none are more or less important than any other. Here are a few you should be aware of:

The Guideline of Equalities (Principle of Correspondence)

'As above, so below; as below, so above.' Everything that happens on your inner plane also happens in your outer world. This paradigm is the major linking agent in the universe, and it is the energy of love-wisdom, and the purpose of this law is to lead the mind back toward the sense of oneness (enlightenment). The thoughts and images we hold in our conscious and subconscious minds will manifest their mirror likenesses in our external circumstances. Our outer world is a mirror of our inner world (and vice versa). Earth is a school for practicing these tools of mind control. This principle enables the phenomenon of Discernment, Intuition, Hunches, etc.

Correspondence enables that which is normally unknowable, to become known to the individual who learns and knows how to use this principle. Some use it in a conscious and deliberate manner while others may not even be aware that they are using this principle. When used knowingly, it enhances the clarity of our vision and enables the mind to penetrate the most secret of secrets, shedding light on many a dark paradox. When used without realizing, we open the door to attracting those things we really didn't want to have!

Correspondence establishes the interconnectedness between all things in the universe and keeps all things relative to each other. There is actually an etheric web that interconnects us all to every aspect of the Universe. This interconnection was known to the adepts and masters of ancient Egypt and has been taught and studied in the mystery schools since ancient times. This substance acts as a medium for the transmission of light, heat, electricity, and gravity. It is non-material in nature and is the substance in which all suns, worlds, and galaxies are suspended in space, time, and change. All of us are intimately connected to all of the above-mentioned events, and to each other, whether or not we realize this. The ethers are where spirit substance is manifesting the beginning of matter. Science refers to this substance as "dark matter" that cannot be seen, touched, smelled, or weighed. Dark matter does not absorb or reflect light and is therefore invisible. It was first discovered on Earth while doing research with the Hubble space telescope. This guideline of correspondence is the process that enables us to bring this 'dark matter' into reality on the earth plane.

The Guideline of Balance

The Universe will immediately counterbalance any impact so that life can be maintained and supported lovingly. The metaphor for this is 'as one door closes another opens.' If you lose a deal, another will come to take its place. The same occurs with customers, jobs, relationships, etc. The Universe is constantly bringing more opportunities forward for us. We have to be alert to see this and not fall into the trap of 'poor, pitiful me' when things don't go our way. Bemoaning a loss creates more loss and activates the Guideline of the Vacuum (see below). Once you grasp this guideline, it is easy to understand that there truly is no such thing as loss in this Divine plan.

Every human has a masculine and feminine aspect to their persona. This is another example of the Guideline of Balance. In fact, in order for conscious creation to occur, we have to activate and utilize both of these aspects. The feminine is the part of us that receives the inspiration and begins the creation through thought, and the masculine is the piece that incorporates the active principle and takes the feminine creation out into the world. The diagram, which most clearly expresses this, is the Dao, the Yin/Yang symbol. The dark half of this sphere is the feminine, magnetic energy, and the light half is the masculine, electric component. In the middle of the dark is a tiny circle of light and in the middle of the light is a tiny circle of dark. Together these parts create a motor, a generator—enabling CREATION!

The Guideline of the Vacuum

Nature abhors a vacuum. When a space is cleared, it absolutely will be filled with the same energy that was there previously, unless it is programmed differently. Clear a space – like energy returns unless you fill it consciously with the positive flow you desire. Here are a few examples that incorporate what we have been discussing:

- Clean out your office [PHYSICAL ACTION] and your desk so that the Universe can fill both up with what you desire [AS ABOVE SO BELOW]. Clutter blocks the flow. This means letting go of everything (clients, deals, paperwork) that is difficult so you can manifest easy, peaceful solutions more quickly [THE PRUNING FACTOR]

- Clean out negative thoughts, guilt, self-deprecation, etc. [MENTAL/EMOTIONAL] so that you can re-program you mind to be more loving—to yourself and to everyone else.

Remember, the definition of insanity is doing the same thing over and over, expecting a different outcome. Unless you fill the empty space you created with what you desire, you will find the truth behind this definition!

The Guideline of Non-Attachment

When you think you know more than God, you are experiencing the ultimate of conceit. The Universe will always give us more than we could possibly have imagined in response to our requests. When we become attached to anything we limit the flow, and since God's answer to every question is always yes, we will receive what we expect. But this guideline doesn't stop here. We are not supposed to be attached to anything. Not our money, not our stuff, not our lover, not our life, nothing. As soon as we are attached, we open the door to fear, and this blocks everything. These attachments weigh us down. They lower our frequency and limit our thinking and creative ability. They also are the underlayment of most fear, because as soon as we become attached to something, we believe that there is a way that we might lose it. This is an illusion, of course, but difficult to see once attachment has taken place.

The Guideline of Order

Everything, if left to its own devices will always be in Divine order. The Universe wants you to be successful and have it all. If you follow the Guideline of Non-Attachment you can't fail! This Universe and all like it are created on a beautiful mathematic scale. We have yet to discover either the smallest component or the largest of it, but scientists have found that even what looks like chaos is actually ordered (chaos theory).

The Guideline of Rhythm

Everything flows – in and out, ebb and flow, the pendulum swing manifests in everything. Only in the ebb can energy be redefined to express in a new and higher way, creating a new flow. All of life has a cycle, just like nature and everything else. Don't get discouraged when the things you desire to manifest aren't flowing in all of the time. Use your time wisely and keep your attitude positive. Using precious time to bitch about the things you aren't getting makes a lot less sense than using your precious energy towards seeing what you can create right now in the present moment. Not only that, but as we have already discovered, you get more of what you think and talk about, so bitching just creates more of the same to complain about! Remember what it says in Ecclesiastes, 'to everything there is a season and a time for every purpose under heaven.' Enjoy when you are in the flow. Move with it, but when the ebb time comes, honor that as well. This is the perfect time for planning, doing your vision quests, planting the seeds that will produce when the rhythm shifts once more.

A beautiful example of this principle is the astrological concept of Mercury Retrograde. Three or four times a year, the planet Mercury will appear to be moving backwards in the sky. Watchers throughout the ages have noted this phenomenon and written about it. It is considered to be a time where there are problematic issues relating to communication and transportation, not a good time to sign a contract or make big decisions or purchases, especially as they might relate to either communication or transportation. What this period is good for is anything that starts with 're': rest, review, research, replay, etc. This is a perfect time to feel the rhythm of the Universe in your life. Use it to your advantage and don't push the river. Clear out everything that doesn't serve you anymore. If you haven't used it in a year or two, find a new owner for it!

The Guideline of Giving and Receiving

As we give, so will energy return to us. When you give freely, you will receive freely; give cautiously, receive cautiously. Always provide more to others than what they ask for or expect. If you fail to follow this guideline, you will block the flow of energy completely. Even down to little things, pay attention! If someone gives you a compliment, for example, and you don't receive it graciously, you have violated this rule and interrupted the flow. It sounds silly, but this applies at every level, from saying 'thank you' to a compliment, to allowing a friend to pay for your coffee, to actually charging for the healing work you do on another. It's all about the flow. This is the guideline that underlies the concept of tithing. Returning a portion of what you receive keeps the flow going, opening the door for more receiving. Don't do this with an attachment to getting something in return, however, because that would violate the Guideline of Non-Attachment. The energy in the Universe is constantly moving, like the breath—in and out. She gives to us with her exhale. We receive and return the energy with our own exhalation.

The Guideline of Patterns

Any habit or pattern tends to reassert itself over time unless we break the pattern by doing something different. As mentioned before, one definition of insanity is doing the same thing over and over, expecting a different outcome. Some patterns are positive and serve us well, so this law calls forth discernment. Examine the patterns in your life to see which ones are working for you and which ones aren't, then release the ones which hold you back and replace them with new ones which assist you in moving in the direction of your choice!

All life on Earth is created in patterns. Living things follow a mathematical sequence called the Fibonacci sequence. We live in a Universe of order. As we raise our frequency to the point of Ascension, we shift our pattern in this mathematical sequence to the larger spectrum, the Golden Mean.

The Guideline of Non-Intervention

It's not our job to interfere or correct what we see as harmful behavior. In fact, calling a behavior harmful is actually a judgment, and is out of alignment with the Guideline of No Judgments. We are to work in our own reality only, for that is the only thing we can really change or control. You can't fix anybody or anything except yourself, so it isn't appropriate to give advice unless it is requested. One of the lessons we come here to learn is that we are supposed to figure out for ourselves which choices serve us and which ones don't. We learn through sticks and carrots. The carrots taste good and feed us well. The sticks are painful and generate aversion.

You will have tons more time and energy if you only worry about and work on your own 'stuff' and leave other people to work on theirs! As you shift and change, you will find that everything around you does as well!

The Guideline of Integrity

Only when we are honest with ourselves can we be honest with another. The first thing you must do is to figure out what is true for YOU. Then stay in alignment with your truth at all times. People constantly ask me, "How can I know what my truth is?" My answer is that if you have to ask whether this or that is your truth, then you haven't found it. Truth is singular. It leaves no room for doubt. Integrity is actually the purity of your intent, and when you stay in alignment with that purity, you can never go wrong.

The Guideline of Divine Flow

When we live in the present moment, centered in love, all flows well. The present moment is all there is. It doesn't serve you to worry about the past or the future, rather just trust that the Universe will provide, and according to the Law of Attraction, of course it will. Keep in mind that the flow becomes obstructed when any of these guidelines is ignored. After all, this is the Planet of Free Choice (see the next guideline), and we have the option at every turn to choose out of alignment with our highest good.

The Guideline of Free Will

We have the right, authority, and power to choose our direction. If you don't like what you are doing, STOP DOING IT! Find something else. There is always another choice. In fact, we each have an unlimited supply of 'do-over's'. You have free will as long as you surrender to what is for the highest and best good of all, not just for you. Issues come when your will is not in alignment with Universal good. Additionally, you can only manifest when your will is in alignment with the will of all those concerned with your manifestation.

The Guideline of No Judgments

Universal Spirit does not judge us. Our judgments attract judgments in equal measure. Start with yourself always! QUIT JUDGING YOURSELF in any way, good or bad. Then, quit judging others in any way. Everything just is. This includes situations, opportunities, co-workers, customers, management, on and on (See the Guideline of Identity). Loving ourselves and others as they are is honoring of our own path and the path of all other's souls. Loving and accepting people and events without judgment or reservation that creates the space for positive change in this world.

The Guideline of Identity

All experiences and things in our lives are seeking to teach us who we really are, helping us to remember who we really are. When we incarnate, our choices and lessons are obscured for us so that we have to seek—stretch—to remember why we are here. Some of us never do. Our true identity is that of creator of our own reality—god. Make no mistake!

The Guideline of Group Endeavor

When two or three or more are gathered together in my name, etc., this is also called the Rule of Collective Energy. Teamwork will always speed up the process. Consider all who are involved in the things you desire and find ways to use the skills and abilities of each to the best good of the whole. Involve everyone as a member of your team, and you will find not only that the manifesting happens more quickly, but the people around you grow through the process as well.

The Guideline of Intention

What you intend to happen is what will happen. Then, energy must follow intention for manifestation to occur. Energy that follows intent always results in creation. Therefore, get clear on what you want, because that is what you will create. It is equally important to get clear on any fear thoughts you have around your goal because they are the "silent saboteurs" of your efforts. You can't move past these blocks unless you are aware of them!

The Guideline of No Expectation

Since energy follows thought, we move toward but not beyond

what we can imagine. What we assume, expect or believe colors and creates our experience. By changing our expectations, we change our experience of every aspect of life. When you expand the box of your preconceived limitations, you add additional colors to your palette, and your painting becomes more beautiful and dynamic. Additionally, expectations lead to disappointment. The only time you will be disappointed is when you expect something or are attached to a particular outcome.

Using These Guidelines

The material in this chapter has been understandably intense, but necessary. Had we been made aware of these guidelines earlier in our lives, perhaps things might have been different and enlightenment progressed more quickly. Who knows? Each of these guidelines will be explored in more detail as we continue to learn about the process of manifesting. Each, in its own way, is your friend, your 'virtual assistant'. Hire your cosmic helper to make your dreams a reality.

Take each of the guidelines, one by one. Make a chart to show how each one applies to your life today. Are you in alignment with it, or are you opposed to it. Or, were you even aware of it? Create an entry in your journal documenting where you are with respect to each one. It will be interesting to see how much shifts when you revisit this in six months or a year.

Chapter Thirteen

In the NOW!

The human mind is a powerful machine, and like any machine it should be operated with care and intention. When you aren't paying attention to your work is when you have accidents.

Do you have any idea what is going on in your mind right this very second? Sure, you are reading this book, and of course you are concentrating to make sure you get every word of it. But do you realize that every moment you have hundreds, if not thousands of thoughts flying around inside your head? And believe me, if you are like most people, the majority of these thoughts are judgmental and not in the least in your best interest.

If you want to succeed at manifesting the things you really want, not the things you really don't want, it becomes imperative that you stay cognizant of as many of your thoughts as possible. It's so easy to get distracted. There are so many interesting things that float past us like butterflies! For example, I can turn on my laptop to catch up with my friends on Facebook before I start my business day, and if I am not careful, I look at the clock, and it's lunchtime! I have just wasted four hours of precious time and have no tangible, revenue-producing things to show for it.

It never ceases to amaze me, when I walk through an office and look at what employees have on their computer screens— solitaire games, social networking sites, You Tube—on their employer's time. This is white-collar theft, actually. When you waste your own time, you are stealing from yourself. Scary thought, isn't it?

Even more frightening are those thoughts you think that you are not aware of. These are the guys that sabotage your efforts to manifest. These are the thoughts of negative self-esteem, unworthiness, doubt, and fear. They are the thoughts that pull you out of the present moment. They set you up for worry about the future—what might happen. They also invoke guilt and pull your consciousness into the past. Either way, you aren't in the present moment. And unless you are there—right here, right now—you can't create. If you keep the TV or radio on while you work or drive, you are constantly flooding your mind with the thoughts of others. This can be especially insidious, because that droning from these devices actually hypnotizes you, and allows the media to access your subconscious mind without your permission. All those words from commercials and song lyrics, not to mention the monologues from newscasters and actors just go straight into your subconscious, which as you know acts like a four year old child, believing every word to be truth. The never-ending stream of pharmaceutical ads prompt your subconscious mind to focus on the very disease they are presuming to be able to cure—effectively creating a market for their drug! This can become quite thought-provoking when you are able to see how each of us can be programmed negatively without even realizing it.

Let me give you a couple of examples of how quickly thoughts are becoming things now:

- I was on my way to dinner with a group of college friends. We were together for a reunion, after many years of going our separate ways. One of them mentioned a friend who lived in the area named Teta. I commented that Teta was an unusual name and my daughter had a friend called Teta. My cell phone rang, and I answered. "Hi Jean," the voice on the other end said. "Remember me? I'm Amanda's friend Teta, and I am calling to see if you would officiate at my wedding next month." We chatted this girl up in a matter of seconds!
- My orchid in the kitchen window was nearing the end of its blooming cycle and I thought to myself, I've never

fertilized this lovely plant—it's time to buy fertilizer and give it a boost after al these years! The next morning, I noticed a new jar of orchid fertilizer on a bench in the garage. It had been left there by a friend. I called and thanked him for being so thoughtful and buying it for me. He said it was actually a gift from his daughter, who had admired my blooming orchid the previous week!

If you are impressed by how quickly these simple manifestations took place, then I am sure you are now actively aware of how important it is to keep any negative thinking out of your reality!

How can you shift your awareness? It takes commitment. It involves waking up. You have to first be in your body. You have to pay attention to exactly how you are feeling and what is going on around you every minute of every day. Turn off the things which distract you—the TV, the radio, your iPod. Understand that it's been proven that it takes twenty-one days to break a habit, so give yourself time for this process to unfold. You might want to set a goal to not watch TV, listen to the radio, read a newspaper, etc. for this period of time. Call it Consciousness Boot Camp.

For twenty-one days, check in on your thoughts and feelings regularly throughout the day. Do it first thing in the morning. I do it even before I drink my morning latte. How am I feeling right now? What was I thinking when I woke up? What do I plan to accomplish today? I find that it helps me to write the answers down. I actually journal these thoughts every morning, because writing them down is a great tool for adding energy to my intent. This keeps me grounded and prepares me for the day ahead.

Repeat this process—every hour in the first days. Later on you can set reminders for two or three times a day. At a minimum, do it first thing in the morning and last thing before you retire for the night. It's really important that you clear away anything that isn't in your highest interest before falling asleep, because when you are sleeping is one of the most powerful times for manifesting. You want to make sure you are manifesting what you truly want!

What if you find negative thoughts when you do this inventory? Guess what? You WILL! You have about seven seconds to erase any thought after you think it before its starting to turn into form. Once upon a time we had a longer grace period, but these days, thoughts become things in the blink of an eye. Can you understand now why it is so important to be cognizant of what you are thinking?

Your mind is your most powerful ally. You can use it to teach your brain to evolve past reptilian fight/flight behavior and into the peaceful mode which enables you to accomplish so much more than you have ever been able to in the past. Mother Nature's goal for us is survival, but to exist in a world where the best we achieve is just getting by is selling ourselves short. If you focus on happiness rather than fear-based thoughts, actions or situations, you start to train your brain to look for more of the same. In turn, this stimulates growth in consciousness as well. Look for goodness and you will find it. When you find it, acknowledge it and look for more.

In one of the concepts of the previous chapter, we learned that energy follows intent and where we put our attention is what we create. Did you fully grasp what this meant? Many people don't understand the difference between intention and attention, and this is a pivotal point in the manifestation process.

First you have to gain clarity around the things you desire to manifest. This is done with intention, which is a yang action. The clearer you are about your desires, the quicker the process works. In order to allow your manifestations to come into reality, you have to be in the present moment and place your attention on what you desire to occur. The second half of the equation is this. Attention is the feminine or yin aspect of the manifestation principle. With this part of the process, you are not doing anything—it's the being, the receptive space that allows you to pull your desired results into reality. All creation must be done in balance—the yin and the yang must both be present in equal proportions if you desire to reap what you sow the way you would like.

Soon, all of this becomes second nature, but in the beginning it may feel like work. However, the rewards for this effort are amazing. You truly have the ability now to have everything you desire.

Claim today as the starting point for your new journey! Take a moment to consciously plan your day. Start with a few deep cleansing breaths, and focus your attention on the present moment. How are you feeling right now? This question is designed to make sure that you are in touch with yourself, in your body and grounded, so give it your best shot—really feel what is going on with YOU.

Now that you are prepared, make a plan for how you would like your day to unfold. Do a sixty second visualization of your day, in the most positive way. For example, I might think...I will have a tasty latte then a shower. My first appointment is a huge success, and I book two good orders. I have a lunch meeting with an old friend who introduces me to a new idea about conscious creation, which helps me on my path. In the afternoon mail I receive a check that enables me to pay off one of my bills. I take a walk through the park and meet someone new who has a lot in common with me. I eat a healthy dinner and read a good book before retiring.

With that I have set my intent to have a pleasant and productive day. I then place my attention of a series of desired outcomes. Nothing too specific, giving the Universe room to make it even better—but I have a plan. I am in charge!

Just surrender your plan to the Cosmic and give thanks that everything you have asked for is yours, and more, in just the perfect proportion, perfect time and perfect way.

Chapter Fourteen

Action – Preparing For Change

It's all about the frequency or energy. If you want to attract anything into your reality, you must first match your vibration to it. In fact, that's really all you ever had to do.

Once you have established clearly where you want to go with your manifestation, you can't just rest on your laurels and expect the Universe to do it all. Well, maybe you can, but if you want to create as quickly as possible, it is in your best interest to take some action. Soon, I will give you an example of the action to take to assist in attracting a romantic partner. Action doesn't have to mean gigantic physical effort on your part. Sometimes it's as easy as visualizing your desires. Remember the guideline—if it's easy for me, it's right for me?

Before you can expect to receive your gifts from conscious creation, you must prepare a place to put them. It's like clearing out space in your closet before a shopping spree or cleaning out the refrigerator before going to the grocery. This is one of the basic rules of Feng Shui. Remember the guideline of the vacuum? Nature abhors a vacuum and will fill it back up quickly.

What are you willing to let go of in order to make room for something new? In today's reality there are some large things to consider. Of course, we can start with the simple ones: clearing clutter, re-arranging furniture and getting rid of clothes we don't wear any more. But now is the time to dig deep inside. The energy of the new reality is supporting our ability to find and release everything that doesn't serve us anymore. This includes, but is not limited to, old inappropriate beliefs, habits and patterns, relationships not based in love, and pain, illness and suffering. Deep inside yourself is where you will find the old gunk that gums up the manifestation process.

Lifetime after lifetime we have created wounds from our reactions to the actions of others. We stored these in our bodies, not just in the physical body although we have done plenty of that, but in the emotional, mental and spiritual bodies as well. These creations have managed to make their way into our very DNA, where we pass them on to our children and our children's children, just like the Bible verse says, "The sins of the fathers are visited upon their sons, unto the seventh generation." Seven is one of those mystical numbers in the Bible. It's a metaphor for "as long as it takes" for someone to assume responsibility and heal the wound.

Wounds from the past are at the source of most of our unhappiness, illness, and pain. Why wouldn't we want to let them go? The answer is crazy but true… We are attached to them. How we feel has become 'familiar' and to feel differently is scary. We get locked into that familiarity so deeply that we don't even remember why we created it in the first place (or when, for that matter.) After all, we managed to survive in the past by developing the very coping techniques that keep us attached to our wounds. This attachment is in violation to one of the guidelines discussed in a previous chapter. This baggage from our past weighs us down and holds us back from the Ascension process. It locks us in to old beliefs and paradigms that don't work for us anymore, and we probably don't even know why we accepted them originally. If these old lessons were inherited from an ancestor or brought in from another lifetime, then for sure they can't consciously make sense in today's world. Once the source of the lesson can be found, it can be examined to see if it fits in your life, and if it doesn't, you can choose to replace it with a new paradigm that does. This last step is important, because if you don't replace it, nature will, and you might be stuck where you were before.

Once you have cleared space for your creation, you need to

align with it. Remember the Guideline of Attraction? In order to magnetize anything to yourself, you must hold within yourself the same frequency. Otherwise you will never attract it, no matter how much work you do. Here is what I suggest. Start by feeling how it feels to already have what you desire. Next, ask the Universe to take your frequency to the level of the manifestation you want to create. Listen to your body as this takes place. By this, I mean listen to your heart. Feel your heartbeat, and you should notice a change as your frequency shifts. It will generally beat faster as the change is taking place, and then will return to normal. At this point give thanks that it is so. Now ask your Higher Self if you are holding the correct frequency of the manifestation. Listen to what you feel in your heart. If you get a 'no', then try the request for frequency change again.

When you have created space for your manifestation, it is time for action. If you fail to take action on your dream, you place yourself in a space of contradiction, because if you are truly clear on what you desire, it only follows that your passion will force you into action. Therefore, if you can't find the energy to take action, you should consider whether you are clear about what you desire. Is it a desire coming from your Higher Self or a need of the ego?

Now is the time to release all those old wounds. This doesn't have to be a difficult process at all. It is just a very necessary one. Here is what I recommend:

Go into a quiet, meditative place. Take a few deep cleansing breaths—in through your nose and out through your mouth. Ask that you be presented with every wound that has not been healed (from every lifetime and from all dimensions) so that you can release and liberate them once and for all. Intend that they all be placed into a big bubble right in front of you. When you feel complete with this it then time for you to take responsibility for your creations, because each of these issues is something that you created. Just say, 'I am sorry that I created each one of you. Please forgive me. I love you. Thank you. I now release you. I liberate you, and I liberate myself.'

You may have to do this exercise many times before you are able to clear away all the blocks you have set up. You might be wondering why this is since we asked that they all be released. Your Higher Self will always prioritize for you and will only help you to clear what you can handle at the time, so that you don't throw yourself into a healing crisis. After you process what you have cleared, more will be presented to you. Sometimes we get little (or large) signals that there is more to be liberated. These can appear as physical pain in the body. If this happens for you, simply put your hand on the place where you feel something to acknowledge it, send love to the spot, and ask your Angels and Guides to present you with all the old wounds associated with this pain and then repeat the process above.

Chapter Fifteen

Forgiveness

The judgments you place on your fellow humans are really just the judgments you have for yourself. Once you grasp this concept and forgive yourself, you free everyone who has become your mirror from having to do that dirty job. They can get on with their life and so can you!

Forgiveness releases the judgments we have stored in our past and erases the associated karmic debt. This brings to mind two very basic questions: why did we make those judgments in the first place, and why have we been so attached to them that we would hold onto those old hurts and resentments for years or even lifetimes? We began the exploration of these questions in the previous chapter, and now we will look more closely at the reasons.

While we lived in duality, the making of judgmental thoughts was the natural outcome of any situation where we were hurt, slighted or did the same to someone else. Those thoughts became things back then just like they do today—things that either materialized as illness, pain or worse, or ones that merely stuck to us or hung in our fields as shapes or thought forms we couldn't see. Basically these judgmental thoughts were tools that reinforced our beliefs that we were separate—from each other or even from Source. They violate the Universal Guideline of No Judgments.

If we hadn't slipped immediately into violation of another guideline—No Attachments, we would have just let these thoughts float away and been done with them, but more often than not, we hung onto every slight, hurt, guilt, remorse or hate and missed the point of the lesson which presented them. It seems to be a basic human characteristic to want to justify an action, and this need to either prove our 'rightness' or receive an apology is a very strong one. So these lessons return to us, and with each reoccurrence, the stakes are raised and the tests get more painful. What if we awakened to the realization that all it ever took was to lay down the sword and walk away from the battle? More often than not we were just attached our 'way'.

My mother used to say, "every time you win an argument, you lose a friend." I don't know if she understood the point she was actually making, but she was teaching me about No Attachments. Every time we become so attached to being right, we make someone else wrong. In an enlightened mind, we would never want to do that, but when we muddle through life half asleep, we forget that 'our brother' is our self, and if we make him/her wrong, we are negating our self; moreover, we are negating God. This is the age-old lesson of The Golden Rule.

The old rules have fallen away as we move into higher levels of consciousness. Humanity and this planet have moved into a place of Unity where they don't fit anymore. Our world is still one of choice, though, so we can certainly keep on doing the same things expecting different outcomes—insanity. Or, we can choose differently this time.

The first step is forgiveness. Start with yourself. What are you judging about yourself? It might be about your physicality (I'm too __ or I'm not __). It might be related to your abilities or accomplishments. There is no order of magnitude in judgment. Just STOP! Forgive yourself, then move back through your memory banks and forgive yourself for everything you have done in the past. Then you can begin forgiving all others you have ever judged or blamed. What they did no longer matters, because the past is gone. It doesn't exist so actions from the past don't exist anymore either. The present moment is all we have. As soon as you can grasp this concept, forgiveness becomes easy. Think of all those old hurts like debts on an accounting ledger. If you feel that there has to be a repayment for each one in order to 'balance the books' you are still living in duality. Look at the ledger your have created for yourself and mark each debt PAID, once and for all! The most incredible miracle follows! As you shed the weight of those old 'debts' you feel lighter. Some will even lose physical pounds as this old gunk falls away, because lack of forgiveness not only holds us back on our path to enlightenment, it weighs us down as well. When you forgive, you let go of fear at the same time, because fear is inextricably tied to judgment. Freedom from fear is the miracle that opens the door to your personal power, allowing you to create the reality you deserve. Realizing this, why would we want to continue on the old path? It didn't serve us in the past, it doesn't serve us now.

Are you having problems with any person in particular as you read these words? Is there someone you just can't bring yourself to forgive because what you believe they did was so despicable that it is beyond your capability to let it go? Let me share another way to look at this. We have soul level contracts with every person we deal with in this life. Some are simple contacts and some are huge, complicated and hard to look at, but nonetheless, they were committed to by both parties prior to incarnation. Why? In order to help each other learn the life lessons we chose for this particular incarnation. So think about it—how much would one soul have to love another to do horrific things in order to assist the other in mastering their goal? If you can get outside the box and look at all of life from this perspective, understanding that this is a grand game, it might make it easier for you.

Forgiveness is critical to clearing the way for conscious creation. It's impossible to be consistent with your manifesting efforts as long as you are holding onto judgment and baggage from your past because this old debris places color onto your thoughts at a subconscious level, eroding your clarity. All this junk acts like ballast on a ship, making it ride lower in the water, slowing it down. As the movement slows, the ship attracts more junk, barnacles, slowing even more, and soon we are not moving in the flow anymore. Eventually we hit the shoals of life and become stuck. We are harder on ourselves than we are on anybody else, so the first place to start forgiving is with 'numero uno'. Letting go of the judgments on ourselves releases a large piece of the ballast.

In the New Testament of the Bible, Jesus tells us to 'love thine enemies and be good to those who would hurt you.' I always inferred this to be about mean people and folks who weren't nice to others. You know, turn the other cheek and all that... But recently, I realized that there was a much broader meaning to those words.

What if we are missing the point in Jesus' message? No doubt there is validity in the people aspect of this teaching, but what if there is more? If we begin to look at how we have been dealing with parts of ourselves, and our lives, as our 'enemies', we open the door for new ways of creating shifts. Carl Jung said, "What we resist persists." And have you ever noticed that the harder you try to change some aspect of your life the worse it gets? I have to believe that Jung was on the right track.

When we fight with the things we perceive are hurting us, we are putting more energy into that area, and according to the Universal Guidelines, where we focus our energy is what we manifest, so it becomes self-defeating work. Even Mother Theresa said that she would never fight or protest for peace, rather she would live peace.

Struggle

Why do we struggle? The obvious answer is because we are human, and that is what humans do, but that is an illusion. The truth is we don't have to struggle. It was never meant to be part of the equation. Struggle is a trap created for us, by us, to keep us from finding our truth. Struggle consumes our energy and blocks us from easily manifesting those things we truly desire.

I sat in the beauty salon recently getting my hair done. Around me I could hear conversations between other clients and their stylists. Struggle must be the new pandemic! Every woman there was talking about areas of dissatisfaction in her life, and much of this centered on struggle, depression or sleep deprivation. I wanted to reach out to each one and say that it doesn't have to be that way, but I figured the response I would receive would be a 'deer in headlights' look and complete disbelief.

The only way I know to end struggle is to surrender to it. It's impossible to play tug of war if nobody is pulling on the other end of the rope. What does it mean to surrender into struggle? Simply let it go. Stop swimming upstream. It's a choice we have to make in order to end the insanity, and we are here on earth to learn about making appropriate choices.

We actually chose individually to create struggle in the first place. It probably started in a very innocent manner. Maybe we just wanted to get ahead at work, or have more stuff, for which we needed more money, and pretty soon we were locked into the game, and caught up in a vortex where we were the unwitting participants. Striving leads us directly into this trap. Rowing our boats upstream is contrary to our highest good.

In a perfect world, we'd get this and just move on, but rarely are we that discriminating. No matter how enlightened we are, struggle lurks around every corner on our journey, and mastery of this lesson goes back to our ability to surrender into it. When we can reach the place we sang about as children, "Row, row, row your boat. Gently down the stream", we don't have to be encumbered with it any more. It's at that point where we can remember the rest of the song—'life is but a dream.' We've been sharing the truth with our children for generations. Now is the time for us to listen to what we are saying, because we always teach what we need to learn.

Why, then, do we continue to deal with struggle? What's the payoff? Perhaps it is the addiction to the drama of it all. There is a certain exhilaration we get with the highs and lows involved. When we throw stimulants like caffeine into this mix, it just exacerbates the issue.

Another reason could be that we have old, archetypal beliefs that we HAVE to struggle. The basic underlying paradigm is that we must struggle in order to earn God's love. This lesson is taught by every dogma, and most of us learn it as truth at an early age. It extrapolates out into other beliefs such as 'we have to work hard in order to succeed' and 'if it is too easy it can't possibly be right'. Nothing could be farther from the truth. All Universal Guidelines point to the path of least resistance as the only way. The Cosmic supports us with flow, and when we move with it, all we require is brought to us. By struggling, we slow the process of conscious creation and rob ourselves of health and happiness.

Most of us have areas of struggle somewhere in our lives. For some people it is finances, for others, it has to do with relationships. How many of us are dissatisfied with our weight? Too much? Too little? And how do we deal with these areas of discontent? Generally we try harder to change them. Work more, get therapy, diet and exercise, and it goes on and on.

Once again, I offer my mantra as your new truth. 'If it's easy for me, it's right for me.' This is the truth that will set you free from the trap of struggle. When life isn't flowing easily, take notice! Stop, take a deep breath and ask the Universe to help you. Let go and Let God. Very soon, if you pay attention, you will be shown another way, an easier solution.

Here are some ideas to assist each of us in releasing struggle and attaining our goals. Start with blessing the area of your life where you desire a change. Bless and love your body exactly as it is and allow it to support you as you find ways to move into better health. Bless and honor each of your bills as you write the check to pay them—honoring the fact that you have money to pay toward the debt. Give thanks for the blessings you have received. As for relationships, call up one or two of your friends and tell them how honored you are to have them in your life. Even better, actually write them a note or send a card! Too few people use the mail anymore—we get by with email or social media, but it brings such joy to receive a personal note in your mailbox, doesn't it? If you want to attract love into your life, you must give love. Find a way to give some love to someone today. Maybe just a kind word to a stranger, but even better if you can go out of your way to do something nice. Perhaps visit an older person who might be lonely, or maybe offer to assist one of your co-workers with a project they have been working too hard on.

We have many tools already to help us to create what we want in our lives. Most of them tell us that we should give thanks that we already have the things we desire to create. I propose that your manifestations will come even more rapidly if you also "love your enemy" and honor your life as it is today as well.

Stuck?

Sometimes I just feel stuck—like I am frozen in a block of ice. It's an interesting metaphor, actually. I can see out, but just can't move. My mind is active. I am thinking, planning, conniving even, but that's as far as it gets. How can I thaw the ice so that I can step out of the frozen prison I have created?

First, I have to generate some heat. Well, if everything is energy, as I believe it to be, then all these thoughts are energy, and energy can create heat. So why, if I have been generating so many thoughts, am I still paralyzed? If the thoughts stay trapped inside the mind they fail to achieve motion, and it is the movement of our thoughts that generates the energy, the heat. One of my friends said recently, "The longest distance in the world is the 18 inches between the head and the heart." The obvious place to move your thoughts then is to the heart. This simple step jumpstarts the process of generating the heat necessary to melt the ice that is holding you in old energy that no longer serves you. Then you can get moving forward on a path to productivity. It's like a Rube Goldberg experiment where the ball drops into the spoon, which knocks the dominoes over, etc.

The metaphysical guideline that explains this is 'energy follows intent'. As we move into higher consciousness, we are called to shift from judgment to discernment. Judgment is head-centered thinking that keeps us stuck. It is in direct opposition to surrender. Discernment is simply judgment that is tempered by the heart. It creates the heat to fuel our forward movement.

Part of what created the big block of ice was judgment of me! Every time I allowed myself to think 'I'm not good enough to…', 'what if this doesn't work', or 'if I do it they might think…' the temperature dropped another degree or two, and I was trapped even deeper inside my icy prison.

I am ready for a spring thaw. This long hard winter of my discontent has passed! I now give myself permission to be free. I release all thoughts that would be limiting. I forgive myself for every thought, word or deed I feel guilty about. I also forgive myself for everything I should have done but forgot to. I now take each idea as it comes into my consciousness and move it into my heart. What does this mean? I allow the heart to examine my thoughts to find the relevance of each one to the rest of the world—how is this idea going to affect anyone or everyone else? What is the potential impact of it? No longer am I limiting my thoughts to my little world. As I look more and more outside myself, I generate more and more energy. This energy not only melts the ice that has held me motionless, but it also fuels my forward progress.

By this point, I expect that you are ready to move forward into the field of potential with a clean slate for creation. In order to have this, it is important that you forgive everyone and every-thing you perceive has ever done you any harm. This can be a rewarding, albeit daunting task. Here is what I suggest:

- Start by decades and review your past. It helps to use pen and paper to do this. Create a linear timeline from birth to the present and divide the line into 10 year increments. Label as many milestones as you can remember, at least one per year. It might be helpful to start now and work backwards.

- Once you have your timeline, examine each year and try to remember any and every one who hurt your feelings, who made you feel "wrong" or who physically or emotionally wounded you. Take your time. Take as much time as you need, because this may be one of the most important exercises you ever do.

- For each person you find, forgive them. Know that whatever happened was a lesson on your path, that it is over and done and doesn't exist anymore. Forgive them ALL. Here is a quick formula for success: take a blank sheet of paper, date it and write "Today is a blank slate for my conscious creation." Then list five things that you are grateful for, and take a moment to write why. Next, write a paragraph of your perfect life, describing everything you desire as though you already have it. Finally, ask your Higher Power to help you by listing three things you need help with. Close by writing, "I now release all doubt and fear and trust that all will be taken care of in a perfect way, and I am grateful." You can then write, "I'm a perfect magnet for love, money, success and much, much more!"

Here is another exercise that will help you to stay in the flow of life so that you don't continue to attract ballast and barnacles that only generate more struggles:

Imagine yourself to be a fishing cork floating in a stream. Notice how you bobble and drift in harmony with the current of the water. Now, see yourself moving downstream, and notice the stones, eddies, shoals and logs as you pass them by. Your 'cork self' isn't attached to anything, because the surface is smooth. If you bump up against an immovable object, the water just pushes you on and soon you are free once more— all done by the flow, not through any effort of your own. Continue this visualization for a few minutes. Do it several times during the day. This exercise has the ability to train your subconscious mind to stay in the flow, not allowing you to stick to anything outside yourself.

Chapter Sixteen

Emotions – The Fuel of Creation

If you knew how important your feelings and emotions are to conscious creation, you would be more aware of them. In order to do THAT, you have to be present in your body.

There is something going on, and we just don't get it. We miss out on huge hunks of time and this leaves us thinking that someone else's reality is not valid, because we don't remember what they said while we were 'checked out'. This is what happens when we aren't present in our physical bodies. We signed up for this journey in these physical bodies on this planet, and then almost immediately many of us found our choice to be a little bit more uncomfortable than we thought it would be. Much of this discomfort is due to those pesky feelings and emotions. When we are in Spirit, we don't 'feel' or 'emote'. Again—why we picked to come here!

Emotions and feelings are key components in the manifestation process. They play different roles, depending on how we use them. *A Course In Miracles* tells us that there are only two true emotions, love and fear, and that anything that is not love is actually fear. Fear is a huge block impacting how quickly we are able to get what we want in our lives. Fear has the ability to masquerade so it can't be easily recognized and hide in the dark recesses where we don't always think to look. We can sweep it out of one area of our life only to find it popping up in another if the doors to that room weren't securely shut. There it will wreak havoc and block our intentions once more. So let's first look at the faces of fear, and then we shall look at the aspects of love.

If fear is anything that is not love, it can be seen in anger, resentment, judgment, guilt, anxiety, hate, control, shame, bitterness—even gossip is a form of fear. If your desire is to create perfect health but you have stored old wounds and bitterness inside your body, you stand a good chance of manifesting illness, even disease instead. If you truly want a healthy, loving relationship but you feel shame or judge yourself in ANY way, you will likely attract a partner who will judge you and magnify your shame.

Most often, the face of fear, which stops the manifestation process, is doubt. In order for the Universe to provide for us, we must be absolute in our certainty that it will. Trust is a huge component here, but because we have been taught that we must be 'self-sufficient', we have a hard time asking for something and then trusting that without our having to do anything further, it will miraculously appear.

Many years ago, when I began to study alternative healing and kinesiology, I realized the power of muscle testing and allowing the body, which will never lie, to show me what the truth was. What I neglected to notice was that the truth that was made apparent with muscle testing was what was true for the present moment, for the person being tested alone. I took this new tool and ran with it—testing everything I could think of, just to see what answers I might receive. In the beginning I got lots of great answers, perhaps because I was asking questions that were relative to the here and now. But soon, I fell into the trap of asking about the future, or about other people and other things that were none of my business. My ego was having a field day! What a sense of power to think one can read another's mind or predict the future, which hasn't even been scripted yet.

What I totally forgot was that everyone, moment by moment, is consciously creating the future and it's impossible to predict it at this point. The fruits of my labors became my downfall, as I continued to test everything. Should I do this? Should I buy that? Is the stock market going to increase today? Will so-and-so call me? Is he in love with me? Will we get married? On and on it went; until I found myself muscle testing almost every minute of the day. It was an addiction, and it was one of the hardest habits I ever had to break.

One day I realized what was happening. Every time I tested to see if something was going to happen or not, I actually DOUBTED my ability to create the outcome I desired. This was blocking my ability to manifest at a huge level. I wondered why I just wasn't getting the things I wanted. I was actually blocking myself. Deeper than this, even, as I doubted, I also started the creation process of those things I imagined when I questioned that my positive creation would appear—a self-fulfilling prophecy, so to speak.

There are several words in the English language that act as clues, if we pay attention to them, that we are interfering with the manifestation process. Should is one such word. This word illuminates the fact that we are operating from victim mentality and looking outside ourselves for answers. When we do this we move our energy from the present moment into a place of fear. We move out of love and into a space where we can't consciously create our reality. It is important to pay attention to our own language, because as Florence Scovil Shinn told us almost a century ago, 'your word is your wand.'

Should is derived from an old English word meaning obliged to or ought to. Here is more of what the dictionary says about it: 1—used in auxiliary function to express condition 2—used in auxiliary function to express obligation, propriety, or expediency 3—used in auxiliary function to express futurity from a point of view in the past. But these definitions don't tell us what happens when we use it as our spoken or written word. There is no way to define the level of disempowerment this word creates.

Anytime you hear this word from a source outside your mind, it is also a clue that you are not in your power center, and you are potentially giving your power away. Our Angels and Guides only teach us with 'gentle nudges'. They NEVER tell us what to do.

This would be in violation of our free will. If you are hearing messages that involve the word should, ask where they are coming from. Ask if they are from Source, from the Light.

Another form of disempowerment comes from hope. Many of us have been raised to believe that hope was a positive thing to do, but this is far from correct. When we sit in a place of hope, rather than trust, we are stuck. Hope puts us into doubt, and nothing gets created in that space. The positive alternative to hope is faith.

Today is a perfect day for you clear away disempowering language from your vocabulary. Set your intention to be aware of the word should as soon as, or preferably before, you utter it. Keep your attention focused on your words.

Next, set your intention to look inside yourself for your answers. Keep your attention in the present and watch to see how many times you are tempted to ask someone else for their opinion on something that concerns just you. Don't go there! When you feel the need to ask someone for their opinion, you give away your power to them and set up the vibration of doubt. This blocks your manifestation progress and it's imperative that you consider eliminating this behavior. This is one of those 'one day at a time' goals. Most of us have been getting input from others about way too many aspects of our daily lives. Remember, the opinion of anyone else is colored by their reality, and probably isn't in your highest interest anyway.

Finally, lose hope. Let yourself be motivated by the knowledge that everything you desire is yours already. If it is for your highest good, it manifests quickly when you trust that it is so. Allow your faith to lead you quickly to everything you desire.

Now you are ready to spend time here on planet earth. Come into your body completely. Ground your energy fully into the core of the earth. Allow your emotions to work for you as you manifest those things you truly desire.

Chapter Seventeen

Patience

Spiritual impatience actually slows your progress. What you fail to realize is the complexity of 'the big picture'. Because everything is interrelated, much needs to take place outside of your knowledge, and until all the pieces are in place, the changes you desire can't take place. When you try to rush the process, chaos ensues.

Lessons come to me on a regular basis. Life provides plenty of clues that should make me take notice, but generally it takes a 2 by 4 against my head to get my attention. After about the third painful reminder, I will usually start to realize that something important is taking place.

It started with the ants. They first appeared in the kitchen a few at a time. Then several showed up in the bathroom. Next about a dozen started marching across my desk. The back deck on my house was being replaced with a much needed, larger, sturdier version, and when the contractor pulled away the cedar siding to prepare to bolt it to the house, a literal army of the miniature workers swarmed out from behind it. Gross!

I asked my friend Dell, who understands nature better than I, what ants mean when they appear like this and she replied, "Who in your household needs to learn about patience?" That would be me. I was fed up with the work ethic of the contractor, tired of waiting for changes in my career, and pushing hard to manifest success for a conference and an upcoming class. Too hard, actually. But it didn't become clear with the ants or even the conference that wasn't as well attended as I had hoped. It took that proverbial broadside slap from the Universe for me to 'get it'. I was at the memorial service for a friend's father who passed away recently, listening to the eulogy being given by the minister.

I felt like he was speaking directly to me when he quoted a verse from Psalm 27 – 'Wait upon the Lord.'

All the hurrying and pushing we do doesn't make the perfect result happen. What we generally get when we do this is what we are able to create by ourselves, not what we might have manifested if we allowed the Divine Plan to unfold. I alone limit myself. Nobody else has the power to do that, and I do it by settling for mortal creation rather than being patient and waiting for the Lord to provide. The key word here is settling. We were never meant to settle for less than what we truly wanted. We were never meant to compromise either. Unless each interaction is a win-win for all involved, balance is lost. Think back to the Balance Guideline. It just doesn't work, and the Universe will seek to correct the imbalance. If we aren't expecting the correction, it can feel as unsettling as it does when the stock market does it!

Impatience begins in our head, so in order to find patience we must first clear our mind of the constant chatter that continuously tells us we must hurry and eagerly provides a long list of things that must be done RIGHT NOW. We easily become deluded into believing that this is real. Stress builds up as we face the ever-growing mountain of stuff to do and quickly we lose track of two important concepts—our priorities and the truth (which is that nothing truly has to be done, ever).

It's amazing how quickly we can be distracted and pulled off our direction and away from those principles and core values that are our truth. There is a Divine Plan to the Universe, however chaotic it might appear. Quantum physicists have proven that there is order, even in chaos. Therefore when times appear to get stressful, it's the perfect opportunity to simply stop and wait for that plan to unfold (or perhaps just catch up to us). As with everything else, it's about choice. You can choose to struggle to achieve your goals, or you can listen to the ancient words from the psalmist and 'wait upon the Lord'. My experience has shown repeatedly that if I will stop and wait, I will be shown a better, easier way, and it will be one that is for the highest good of all rather than just for me.

It isn't always easy for those of us who are used to being in control and competition to surrender to that Divine Plan and accept that there is plenty for all of us. We don't have to 'get there' first in order to be taken care of. If we allow it, everyone will be. Wait patiently and see what happens.

Patience is extremely important in the creation process. One of our first steps is clearing space for our manifestations to take place, right? This means that we have to let go of the things that no longer serve us, and part of this process requires taking an inventory of what we have so that we can know what to keep and what to release.

Fear is the main block on forward progress and higher consciousness, so the number one thing on my 'release list' this year was letting go of all fear. We have to be careful what we ask for, because we just might get it. I set the intent to release ALL fear from my life, and the Universe winked and said 'Woohoo.'

Just like what happens when a demolition crew takes down a building—if the foundation is destroyed, the entire edifice comes toppling down. So if fear has been a major component in the foundation of one's reality, if it is removed, guess what happens? It can turn a peaceful life into a train wreck! My back began to hurt, my legs ached, my knees refused to bend, and unexpected large bills cropped up to sabotage my savings account!

What's the lesson here? When a structure is repaired, first the foundation must be shored up before removing big pieces to replace them. How can this be accomplished? First, ask your Angels of the Highest Light to remove your negativity and fear a little at a time—by the teaspoon if necessary. It is very tempting to ask that it be taken away all at once, but on doing that you risk turning your reality upside down. More is not always better. Next, fill in the gaps with new, more positive behaviors. Patience, grasshopper!

One example of fear in my life was the manifestation of criticism, of others and of me. This was a deep-seated issue, and I didn't realize how deep until I decided to change the behavior. When I brought this recurring pattern up for clearing, I noticed that it got worse as I tried to stop it. For more on this read the chapter on Creating Healing! I opted to replace this negative behavior with a compliment every time I was tempted to snipe at someone else or think less of myself. In the cases where I just couldn't come up with something nice to say, I would just express gratitude. Before I knew it, I was back on track and moving forward toward my goals—easily, peacefully and harmoniously!

Relax and Release

The way to find patience is to relax and give up control. Here are some things you can try to help you to release the attachment to a particular outcome, especially if that attachment is to a timeframe:

- Take a look at what's going on in your life right now.
- Find three things you are expecting to happen on your timeline.
- What would be the worst thing that might occur if your time criterion wasn't met?
- What could you do to modify this occurrence by changing something that IS within your purview?
- How did you affect this situation that's been causing you stress with a simple shift?
- Examine all three things on your list and make the appropriate change in your expectations now.

Chapter Eighteen

Creating A Relationship

In earlier times, when you were primarily Light, you carried both aspects—male and female—in balance, and you were able to manifest more quickly and easily. Until you return to that level of balance, you will find that your ability to do high alchemy is enhanced when you work in relationship with another who balances your energy.

So, you say, 'I am putting all my attention on finding a new partner. I think about this day and night, but he or she never shows up. What am I doing wrong?' Your answer lies in your focus. If your awareness is that you are missing this partner from your life, then the picture you are showing to the Universe is one where you are standing in a lovely garden and there is a gray hole standing right next to you where your partner should be...And the Universe says, 'Yes, it is so.'

Let's change this picture to enable the conscious creation you desire. See yourself in that garden working side-by-side with your partner. In this new picture, we see only your backs as the two of you diligently fertilize, weed and plant together, having fun and enjoying each other's company! We can't tell from this picture what your partner looks like because his/her back is toward us. What we see is two people in harmony with one another, having fun. And the Universe says, 'Yes.'

You have your picture now, but before you can attract this wonderful partner, you have to go back to the Universal Guidelines we discussed earlier. Like attracts like, so if you want to create a partner who is healthy, supportive, generous, kind and loving you must first find these attributes within yourself. You can only create what you already are. The key to doing this is finding and releasing ALL the old wounds, stored programming and judgments in yourself, before you ask to have what you desire—otherwise you will manifest a mirror of yourself, complete with all your own issues to show you what you need to heal. Oops!

Our Higher Self has a wonderful and loving way to bring all our warts and scars to the surface for healing and release. I call it the 'Carrot and Stick' method. Carrots are the gentle clues that we have an old wound requiring attention. These clues come to us in meditation, quiet time and our dreams. The problem is getting our attention! How much quiet time do you allow yourself? Most of us have our iPods in our ears or keep a constant drone from a TV or the computer that fills our heads and blocks the input from that 'still, small voice within'. If you are lucky enough to catch the message from within and are serious about clearing the way for conscious creation, you can take these messages to heart and let them go. It's a fairly simple process. Put your attention on the pain or the hurt you need to let go and say, 'I am sorry I created you. Please forgive me. I love you. I release you. Thank you.'

The Stick gets us when we ignore the Carrot messages. If we choose not to listen (notice I use the word choose because this is all about free will, and we can ignore easily and the lesson will just slip back into our subconscious for a while), the next time the lesson surfaces, it will try to gain your attention by creating pain, physical pain somewhere in your body generally. This time the lesson hurts, and every time we ignore it the pain increases—up to and including disease or traumatic 'accidents'. This process goes on and on until we choose to end it by dealing with our wounds, or not.

Here is another example of 'like attracts like': Mary's mother had two failed marriages where the theme was abuse. Mary was the product of the first one. When she grew up and married, she also married an abuser, and when she had enough she divorced him. Time passed and she met Mr. Right. This man was not an abuser. He was kind and loving—everything she always thought she wanted. BUT... Mary carried within herself the energy stamps of abuse she inherited from her mother (who actually inherited them from her mother) and lurking within her subconscious mind was a belief that 'men will hurt me'. Because, as it says in *A Course In Miracles*, 'love brings up everything unlike itself for healing and release,' Mary's new partner will honor her beliefs. This man, who before Mary, wouldn't have hurt anyone, will say 'yes' to her subconscious mind. No sooner than they actually committed to each other, he began to abuse her in honor of her thoughts! This happens more often than you can imagine. Mary will continue to repeat this pattern relationship after relationship until she wakes up and lets the old, inherited wound go.

Change starts within. Before you embark on a quest to create the perfect love in your life, find the love for yourself. The first relationship you must create is the one with yourself. Clear away all inappropriate beliefs that aren't working for you. How do you find them? Start back at awareness and look at the relationship areas that aren't producing the results you really want. Change your thoughts and you will change your life! Use the I AM statement I AM Self-Love.

Many books have been written teaching conscious creation. They all say to visualize and get clear on what you want, but I am presenting a different take on this. Of course it is important to visualize. Thoughts create things. And without clarity, our thoughts create chaos. This technique of visualizing the action you want with the actors facing away is new. Second, is remembering that you can only create what you are. This aspect of clarity says that you have to get healthy in order to receive a healthy partner. Remember, it is important to fill up the hole where you previously placed your attention on what you were missing with something that is actively participating with you in doing something that elevates your feelings to joy, bliss and love. Active participation is the key!

At this point, you are either IN a relationship or you desire to create one. If neither is the case, you can go on now to the next chapter. Let's examine each situation separately:

- If you are IN a relationship, take a moment and evaluate how you might be able to make it better. Visualize the areas of your relationship that work really well and give thanks for them. What aspects could use a little touch-up (or a major overhaul)? Generally our ego will take us straight to the things our 'other half' doesn't do the way we would like. The only person in a relationship you can change is YOU. So start praising your partner every time they come close to doing the things you like, rather than telling them what move you want them to make next. It's tried and true behavior modification—not manipulation, and it works. All of us respond so much better to praise than punishment.

- If you are looking for a relationship, visualize yourself and your partner having fun doing something fulfilling and give thanks that you already have Mr / Ms Right in your life.

Chapter Nineteen

Creating Success

If you knew how powerful you really are, you would never worry about being successful at anything. You would simply create it! Why don't you?

What does success mean to you? How do you define it? In which area of your life are you falling short of success, and where do you feel you have achieved it? Success means different things to different people. One of the interesting trends I have noticed in my research is how many people are willing to settle for just getting by and think that equals success. If the proverbial wolf isn't at the door, then this must be success. That is scary. When we settle for less that we truly desire, we are actually compromising.

Compromise is something that sets up wounds for us to clear. I know that most of us were taught that it was the right thing to do, but every instance where all parties in a situation didn't win, then somebody felt pain, and as we have already learned, when one of us hurts, at a deep level all of us hurt. Compromise always creates pain. 50/50 just doesn't cut it. 100/100 is the only healthy way to solve any situation. Success is where all parties receive more than they thought they deserved. It's the Guideline of Three.

In Universal Order, one plus one doesn't equal two. It actually makes three – the sum of the whole is always greater than the sum of the parts. Bet you didn't realize that. So, in order for the creation to be a conscious one, you have to find the higher thought or concept, always.

Why shouldn't we have it all in every area of our lives? I believe that is our birth right, but somewhere along the way, many of us have been taught otherwise. Deeply held beliefs and myths have told us that we don't deserve this. In some cultures having 'too much' is actually deemed to be a sin.

A common belief I find in many of my clients is 'it isn't appropriate to pick ME first'. This program plays out in several ways, but the one I see most often is that the person lives their life trying to please everyone else. This is the most destructive form of compromise. They put their dreams and plans on hold while they live the lives that they think everyone else expects of them.

Perhaps you wonder why I would attract so many clients with the same issue—probably because it is one of my own deeply held programs! I began playing this game when I was very young. I allowed my dad to tell me how to behave and my mom to tell me what I was supposed to aspire to. Mom wanted me to play the piano and dance ballet. Those were two easy tasks for me to do. I enjoyed both of them, but neither was something I dreamed about, and both are skills that require practice in order to develop proficiency. While both gave me pleasure, that pleasure didn't outweigh how much I disliked the practice part. Therefore, I was never successful with either. My mom's emphasis on piano was so strong that at age five I walked alone to the home of the local piano teacher to ask if I could study with her. She smiled and told me to come back and ask again when my little hands were big enough to span an octave on the piano. This is the first instance I can remember of striving to overachieve to please my mother.

The pattern continued throughout my life, until my mother passed away, actually. I allowed her to choose my classes and my major in college. I even allowed her to pick the sorority I would join. These were all CHOICES I made (remember—there are no victims).

My dad, on the other hand, wasn't present most of the time, so I strove for success to get his attention. I endured countless hours in the Rainbow Girls order to please him—hating it all the way.

All those years I did what others wanted were years that I never looked inside to see what would really make my heart sing. I just kept "showing up". I continued running this program until I was almost sixty years old! Time after time, I "lost myself" in relationships, jobs, and more.

This story is an example of what happens when we don't understand what is really important to us at the bedrock level, and if we don't know that, then it's impossible to see success when it occurs!

I just shared with you the ramifications of life choices on a surface level, but they run much deeper than the surface. Remember how we learned that every cell of the body has a soul? Well, each of our organs and glands does as well. When we don't live in integrity and authenticity, our organs, glands and cells suffer too. The organ that took the brunt of my compromising behaviors was my pancreas. The soul function of the pancreas is to identify one's true feelings and be able to express them, which in turn makes us feel happy and nurtured. When the pancreas is wounded due to compromise, we get disconnected from our true feelings and can't express them, creating a hunger for more sweetness in life (craving sugar or alcohol to satisfy). Then because the body wants homeostasis, it will recruit other organs or glands to counterbalance the problems, so I ended up with a lot of stress and issues with my lymphatic system to boot.

Manifesting success is really no different than creating the perfect relationship. You will use the exact same tools. Start with awareness. Pick the first area where you desire success. Remember, focus is important so that your energy flows where you are choosing to make a shift. Define what success means to you. One of the major obstacles in achieving success is not knowing what it is—and if you can't define it, you don't realize when you actually have achieved it. Success may look different in different areas of your life, so don't get locked into a single defin-ition. Expand your thoughts about success. Give yourself permission to think BIG. Allow God to have a field day in providing for you more than you could have possibly imagined. Remember, the answer to every prayer is 'yes'!

In order to be abundant one has to be successful, and what we are really looking at here is abundance. Success is energy, and it is a reflection of the energy of love. When we say 'I am in a successful relationship', we don't mean a relationship without ... but a relationship that is rooted in love and in its various qualities such as respect, acceptance and so on. Success means working the way you are 'supposed' to work, and love is what that is built on. Without love there is no success and being able to choose success is being able to choose love. In fact, they are one, and every time that we ask for healthy success, it all comes down to this: I love me, I love the spirit in me, I love the life in me, I love my life, I love life, I love the Creator, and I love the Creation, and I am one in and with this love. Your life is a celebration, so allow it to be a celebration. Believing that this party is real and not a dream is a great step forward. Know that being invited to your celebration is not a mistake. You created it and you deserve it totally.

Chapter Twenty

Creating Money

Money is just another form of energy. It's a reflection of you and what you believe. As humans you have created an entire belief system around it.

Money is the major area of many of our lives where we consistently experience lack. Why is this? Obviously there must be inappropriate beliefs that we are holding onto that are blocking our ability to manifest financial abundance. The first key is to identify these so that we can release them. It sounds simple, but many of the blocking beliefs around money are so deeply hidden within our subconscious minds that we have completely forgotten them and why they were put there to begin with. The second key is to find your passion and allow that to attract and build the financial abundance you crave. Finally, in alignment with the guideline of attraction, you must *become* the energy of money in order to have it flow to you.

Where did these beliefs that we weren't supposed to have wealth originate? There are many sources, but one predominant theme arises from religious dogma and associated greed. How better to fund the coffers of an ideology than to tell the followers that it's sinful to have too much and that a certain amount of all their harvest should be turned over to the 'church' or government? This practice has been going on throughout recorded history and continues successfully today in many factions of society.

Please don't confuse this with the Universal concept of giving and receiving—keeping the flow. Absolutely the Universal Guideline tells us that we should return a portion of what we receive to the good of the 'all'. I interpret this to mean that we should give a portion of our bounty to those who feed us spiritually, who feed our souls. This doesn't necessarily mean to a church or organization, unless we are receiving that level of nurturing from it. On the other hand, the recipient of our tithe might be a massage therapist, a librarian who suggests positive books to support our growth, a teacher, healer, and the list goes on and on.

You have to believe that you are capable of receiving anything that you request from the Universe. What does this mean, exactly? Your energy has to be in alignment with your request. So, if you are looking to manifest money, you have to be aligned with money. No fears can be associated with money; in fact, you must LOVE money in order to attract it! For example, one fear that seems to be common is this: 'I have gotten money before, but it was taken away from me (by an unexpected bill or a loss, for example)'. If you have ever had this thought, it means that you are out of alignment with money. The truth is that there is never any loss in the Universe – the guideline of Balance assures us of this. When you can accept this as your truth, your resonance and vibration then can line up with your desire.

Another aspect of manifesting money has to do our attachment to the ways we expect financial abundance to arrive on our doorstep. The whole paradigm around this as well as the energy of money itself is shifting. If fact, those things that require us to use money are changing. As we begin to look at the world through new filters, our so-called needs are reduced, and the inflow comes in to match this though new channels, such as barter and gifts. It's interesting to watch this in manifestation! Only two centuries ago, we lived from the land. Life was simpler, and much of what we had to get from the outside, we actually did by trading: my eggs for your grain, etc.

For too long, the assumption has been that in order to manifest money, one had to work—work hard. The cycle of hard work to support a lifestyle, with the associated income followed by outflow became the rule. For many life has become a treadmill that is impossible to jump off.

Manifesting money in the new reality requires shifting consciousness to open to the possibility that our assumptions up to this point have been incorrect. It requires letting go of all preconceived notions about money.

The new basic principle is that money follows Joy. It's quite simple actually. If you want to manifest more money, you have to get in alignment with joy in all aspects of your life! No exception. Whoever said that rich people are never happy just didn't know truly wealthy people. Start by examining the life of the richest people in the world—Bill Gates and Warren Buffett are great examples. They are HAPPY! You don't hear about them on the drama circuit, do you? Oprah falls into this category as well, although she seems to have some residual baggage around money beliefs that trip her up from time to time. But, she's more in alignment with the flow than not, so if you notice, she always comes out ahead financially. More often than not, I have to believe that she is happy. Additionally, if she wasn't aligned with abundance, she wouldn't be able to do the work she does for the highest good of all. Oprah is a great example of being in the flow.

The process of creating money works just like it does for creating relationships and success. Get clarity first: what do you desire the money for and what do you plan to do with it. Then ask for it by being grateful that you already have what you require and more, so that the universal response can be yes, yes and yes. Finally, align yourself with the energy of money. How have you felt in the past when you were prosperous? What does it feel like to receive a big check? A gift of money? Even the excitement of winning $250 from a slot machine in Las Vegas! Remember times when you didn't have to think before buying something or spending money for anything you just wanted for no particular reason. Now remember a time when you gave money to someone, just because. How did THAT feel?

As we move deeper into 2012 and higher in consciousness, we find new and different avenues are opening to provide financial abundance to us. In fact, new ways are appearing to provide every type of abundance to us.

Every Wednesday morning at 9AM Eastern Time, an extremely large group of people take fifteen minutes to meditate on receiving some type of abundance in new, different and unexpected ways. They have been doing this for quite a while now with some very interesting results. Some have gotten unexpected sums of money, others have found new people and places to offer their wares and services, even others have found ways to barter so that they receive what they need and someone else gets their desire without money having to change hands.

When someone new hears about this group, the same questions tend to arise…generally something like this: 'It's in the middle of the night where I live' or 'I have to watch my grand-child at that time and I wouldn't be able to concentrate or get still'. Time is an illusion too, so all you have to do is decide to participate. If you can't do it physically, some aspect of your persona—your higher self, for example—WILL do it, and you reap the benefit as if you were sitting still and visioning a cornu-copia of wealth flowing into your lap. You don't have to sign up for this group. Just start doing it. Take the time to put your attention on abundance and your energy will find the energy of this group, and you too will get the benefits of group endeavor.

Create a prosperity desire list for yourself with goals and objectives related to financial success. Every day, take a minute to put your attention on your desire list and surround it with pink light. Pink is the color of love, so you are aligning your prosperity desires with the frequency of love!

Prosperity Mantra
Pronounced: Om Shree Mah-Ha Laksh-Mee-Yei Swah-Ha

Meaning: Om and salutations. I invoke the Great Feminine

Principle of Great Abundance.

Explanation: The energies of water and earth are female. Physical energy is form, and prosperity is energy in form. Calling on the great female presence puts thought into the form of prosperity. The goddess Lakshmiyei personifies our own ability to create wealth and abundance in all forms.

Practice: Write on a card. Chant 108 times each day for 40 days.

Passion Power – Allow your passion to fill your wallet

Are you tired of working in a j-o-b, making money for someone else? Are you appreciated for the work you do? Do you wake every morning, excited about what you do for a living? Unless you can answer 'yes' to these three questions, you have not yet found your passion. And until you begin living in your passion, you will be stuck in the cycle of lack, settling for less than you deserve.

Shifting out of this rut is a fairly straightforward process. There are six basic steps you will need to follow:

- What is your passion? If money was no object, but you still had to work, what would you do—that you could do every day and make your heart sing while you support yourself?
- How much money do you desire and require? Make two lists that reflect monthly amounts. The first list is the require list, and on it, quantify the amount of money you require to meet your current obligations (rent, insurance, car payment, gas, utilities, food, etc.) The second list (mandatory!) quantifies the extra money you desire for fun things like vacations, clothes, movies, lattes, manicure/pedicures etc. Add the two amounts and tell the Universe that this is how much money (or more) you desire to receive for living your passion.
- How much time will you devote? Include the amount of

time you will spend each week doing your passion, plus the amount of time each week you will spend in play, plus the amount of time you commit to rest.

- Do you require any additional training in order to do what will make your heart sing? How much and when can you get it?

- Address your fears about this process. Make a list of all your limiting beliefs about why this can't possibly work for you. Go back over this list and analyze where each of the beliefs originated. Then re-write each one into the positive so that it supports you in doing what you love to do.

- Finally – decide when you are going to start!

We are at an amazing time in the evolution of our consciousness. We have the ability to create everything we desire with our thoughts and our mind. Not only that, but it happens very quickly now as well. Therefore, why would any of us limit ourselves if we don't have to anymore? It is up to each of us to take responsibility for creating what we want, and this passion power process is the first step. We ARE the creation of our reality, and by honoring that and loving it, the Law of Attraction steps in and just keeps giving us more of what we desire.

Chapter Twenty One

Creating Health

Your physical body is one of the most responsive aspects of your reality. Every individual cell in it has a soul that responds to you as the creator. All you have to do is ask, and your cells will do your bidding. You were never intended to age and die. You created that illusion, so take charge of your body now.

The body is the 'bubble of biology' the Soul creates to enable itself to have a physical experience and learn the lessons that can only be learned in this type of vehicle. When we put on these bodies, our first experience is that of being separate, from others and from Source. Of course this is natural, because the lessons of the body are about separation and lack of love, and so it's part of the plan. In a perfect world, we would travel through our life without sickness and pain, but we create these things along the way to assist us in learning our lessons. How better to understand separation and lack of love than to feel disease and pain. Think about it! How do you feel when you are sick? Do you feel all alone? Do you just want to be left alone?

The only person who can heal you is YOU. For centuries, lifetimes even, we have given away our power to others, thinking that they were capable of healing us. We have allowed doctors of all types to practice medicine on our body temples. We have prayed for help to the Cosmic, Angels and Saints when all the while the power has been within us to release the pain of disease and return ourselves to the perfection that is our birth right.

So why has this been hidden from our reality? In fact, it has not. Volumes of information have been published over the centuries providing the instructions that would enable us to heal ourselves. The Master Jesus healed the sick and said, "Everything

I do you can do and more." But we didn't understand what he was telling us.

This morning I had a breakthrough! For two weeks I had experienced severe mid-back pain, and my natural doctor told me it was being caused by gallstones. I went looking to see what they mean energetically—anger and resentment—and started doing energetic clearing work using InnerSpeak in addition to a liver and gallbladder cleanse. Several sessions later, I finally reached the core, that place where I actually had the key to let go of what had created the stones that were slowing my forward progress.

What I found was that the anger and resentment were based in old thoughts and judgments I had made about my own body—that it wasn't doing what I wanted it to when I expected it to and how I thought it should. Every one of those angry thoughts had formed a rock inside me, and it took a year or two of this to reach the level of pain where I would actually pay attention. But these judgmental issues had been building up for years, if not lifetimes. The carrot turned into the stick two weeks ago. Time to get serious about healing myself, I realized.

I woke this morning with an 'Aha' thought! I got the lesson and remembered when I started beating myself up. The funny part is that I didn't realize that this was what I had been doing. I had forgotten one of the most basic principles in metaphysics. I truly didn't understand that I was creating stones with little thoughts. Trust me—if I had, I would have said "erase, erase" immediately!

The back pain left with the realization of my part in the process. There was still tenderness in the gall bladder area, so I did a liver flush to release the residue. I was amazed at the amount of stones I had created and stored in my body—over ninety of them. It actually took three liver flushes before they stopped coming out.

Please don't misunderstand me. I believe that there is a time and a place for modern medicine and traditional doctors. However, if we don't get to the root cause—the thought pattern or belief that was the original source of the mistake that manifested in disease, we will never be able to heal. Drugs and surgery will treat the symptoms, but the underlying wound will remain until it is liberated. And unless it is released, the medical problems will have a tendency to recur. True health involves body, mind AND spirit. Neglecting any one of this triad will mean that blocks in the area of health will have the ability to manifest.

As we move forward in this shift of the ages, it is incumbent upon each of us to find all these wounds at every level and let them go. They don't fit in the new reality, and they will impede our progress to get there. If we are looking at living in Heaven on Earth, we have to allow our bodies to heal and attain perfection as well. As we remember who we always have been, we also remember our Divine Blueprint that will enable us to heal, once and for all time.

These bodies we created to house our souls respond very well to our intentions. We can create anything we desire—this has been shown in every chapter of this book. So why not create for yourself the perfect body? Science has proven that the cells in our bodies replace themselves fairly rapidly. You have an entirely new skin every 6 months—every cell is new and different. Why would you want to create skin with blemishes and wrinkles? What purpose would that serve exactly?

Start by getting really in touch with your own body. Every cell has a soul of its own. This is a holographic universe, and your body is no different. Every cell contains the image of your whole body, right there in the DNA! You can talk to your cells, smile at your cells, even sing to them if you want to. Definitely, the place to start is with sending love to each and every one of them.

Earlier in this book you learned the guidelines by which the Universe operates. One of them taught that when you release one thing, you should replace it with something better. When you released all the old wounds that were programming your body to decay and die, you left some great empty space, the perfect place to plant the thoughts to create the perfect body, don't you think?

Let's talk more about why we came here. Part of our task on earth is to learn about love, and in order to do that we have to experience lack of love. This is why we picked bodies as the tool to give us the illusion of being separate from each other, because if we remembered that we are all one, like we are at Home, how could we feel any lack of love? We borrow our bodies from the earth, from the elements of the earth, carbon, water, etc. So, what are the rules when we borrow something? You are expected to use it and return it and take good care of it while you have it, right? It's the same with our bodies. How many of you ever thought about your body in that way? And when you get ready to return it to the earth when you are done with it, will you give it back in the same condition that it was when you got it, or will you give back something that is old and worn out? My guess is that few of us have taken the same care of these borrowed bodies, as we would have a car borrowed from a friend. It's our duty to create good health for our bodies. It's part of good stewardship. We can start today thinking about how to take care of the body so that we can return it properly. In doing so, we make our time here on the planet easier and happier.

The bottom line here is that thoughts really do become things. In order to have health in every area of our lives, we must flush out all toxic thoughts. This includes judgment in every form—of other people, of life situations and of our self. Another type of toxic thought relates to gossip. Every time you are involved with gossip you have fallen into that judgment trap. Complaining is a third example. Earlier we learned that where we put our awareness is what we manifest, so complaining just keeps us locked into a space of not changing away from the things we

DON'T want.

Since thoughts do become things, the toxic ones will absolutely manifest into reality stuff you really don't want in your life, such as illness, accidents and unexpected loss of money, relationships and material things.

Commit today to clean up your mind, stop all judgment, and cease gossip and judgment in any form. Monitor your thoughts and words and shift the energy if you catch yourself moving into any form of negativity. Remember, it takes twenty-one days to break a habit, so don't judge yourself if you slip along the way.

We tend to lapse into an interesting mental place when we drive our cars. Anger and road rage at other drivers and the choices they make can pull us off our direction, so be particularly aware of this. If you find yourself criticizing the actions of another driver, change that thought to one of love. You will be surprised at how this will make a difference in your energy.

Let's do an exercise. Is there any area in your body where you have a known disease? If not, skip to the next paragraph, but if the answer is yes, let's drill into the issues. Place your attention on the location in your body that is the focus of this appearance of disease. Ask your body to assist you by sharing with you when you thought the thought that created its onset. Become very quiet and listen to your thoughts. What is your body telling you? Take a piece of paper and write the thoughts that come into your mind. Allow the words to flow onto the paper without thinking about grammar or spelling. Clues which might assist you or your medical practitioner in assisting you in creating healing may flow to you in your writing. For sure, it can't hurt!

The second part is to fill your body with Love. Tell the Universe, "I now give to my body all the energy and love that it needs, now and for the future, and so be it!" Now experience what happens. Feel the energy flow into you and infuse you. Stay focused in peace, love and joy!

Chapter Twenty-Two

Accountability

Once you begin to accept that you are accountable for everything in your reality, it only makes sense for you to create more of what you want and less of the rest, right? All the time you spent thinking that it was coming from somewhere or someone else just kept the priceless gems at arm's length. You were never able to reach them, no matter how much you yearned. As soon as you woke up to the fact (that was always true by the way) that you could have anything you wished for, things got much easier and voila—you got them!

Once you realize this beautiful gift of creation you were born with and begin to use it to its fullest advantage, you have to then take responsibility for the things you create. Additionally, you get to take responsibility for being the creator of all you survey.

Humans have the unique ability to observe our circumstances from every angle and make decisions or rationalize based on what we see. Unfortunately, we often forget to do this and get so caught up the in drama that we become focused on a single facet of life and lose sight of any other possibilities. This shrinks our perspective and turns three-dimensional reality into a flat two-dimensional picture. Our power to change and create becomes lost in the landscape. Objectivity is a gift. It is our birth right as a human being. We may be the only species on this planet that has this ability to observe and then reason based on our observation. I say we may be the only species with this gift, because I believe it is possible that the cetaceans (whales and dolphins) have it as well, but since we are unable to communicate with them, we can't know this for sure.

In order to be good stewards of our birth right of objectivity, we must utilize it. Take every opportunity to hone your skills of observation and witnessing. As we release judgment, it becomes easier to see that everything and everyone just 'is', and it follows that we can then look at every situation we encounter more objectively, from every angle. Like a photographer, take a step back and allow your viewfinder to include more information. When you do this, a beautiful thing happens—possibilities and potentials begin to appear. Ideas which might never have occurred to you light up before your eyes. Pandora's Box of creativity unlocks and opens, and you have CHOICES you can make! Life is no longer black and white, but a million shades of gray, layered with more colors than a Pantone color wheel.

Do you remember in school, where you weren't allowed to grade your own quiz or homework? The teacher would tell the class to trade papers, and then she would read the correct answers. In real life it's a bit different. We don't have anyone to review what we are doing and tell us when we get off course. In fact, the more we validate our own actions, the farther off course we can go!

As you play in your choices, it is incumbent upon you to continually check to make sure you are still moving in the direction of your truth. This is a big part of accountability. Set aside time on a regular basis to tune in to your core values. The best way to do this is through a regular practice of prayer or meditation. There is no better source to check in with than your higher self.

Every facet of life shines light on a choice, an opportunity to exercise your free will. After all, that is why we chose to incarnate on this planet this time—to learn lessons involving free will. Don't waste another minute with would, should and could. Practice using this wonderful tool. Use every encounter to look at every possible aspect and every potential choice. Choose wisely! Your destiny depends on you taking responsibility for creating it and making it happen.

For centuries folks who have lived from the land have known

that for the best harvest, it is wise to plant seeds on the dark of the moon. If you believe that every thought is creative (and even if you don't, you should consider this), you can amplify your conscious creation opportunities by planting your intentions on the new moon as well.

The period of time, which occurs the last few days prior to the new moon, is called the balsamic moon. This is your time to vision quest. It's a perfect time to go within and make your plans for the future. Just like the farmer cultivates his soil before planting his crops, this will serve to till your inner landscape and prepare for your manifestations to come. Remember, every answer lies within you, so take time to dig deeply.

Every thought you have is like a tiny seed. You plant it and almost instantly it begins to take root and push up toward the light. Your thoughts create beautiful flowers and tasty fruits and vegetables, but they can also create weeds. Constantly monitor your thoughts so that you allow only what you desire to take root in your garden. If you find a weed, get rid of it by changing the thought pattern that created it. These beautiful plants that have grown from your consciousness now need you to nurture them.

Let's talk about tending this wonderful garden you are building. Just like little children need healthy food and love to thrive, your garden of consciousness requires that you nurture it as well. In order to allow your thoughts to manifest into reality quickly, feed them with trust and energy. The energy that provides the best nutrition for your thought garden is love. Your feelings and emotions are the fertilizer that supports high yield, so add copious quantities of enthusiasm, excitement and joy and your harvest will be bountiful soon.

Share the fruits of your garden with others, and you will receive even more blessings. The Universal Law of Giving and Receiving tells us that as we sow so shall we reap, so be generous with what you harvest. This is accountability, the third component in the manifestation process.

Let's examine a recently planted seed. Think of a project you have wanted to start or might have actually just begun. How can you nurture this seed so that it can climb to maturity in the perfect time? Your fertilizer is love, so allow yourself to only think positive thoughts about your desired outcome. When you catch yourself doubting, change the thought to something more supporting. If you can't come up with a better alternative, try getting quiet and asking your heavenly helpers to assist you. Let go of any attachment to an outcome, then open yourself to receive, allowing the Cosmic to bring everything to you in the perfect way.

Chapter Twenty-Three

Wonder VS Wondering

Do you remember when you were very young, you believed in the
Tooth Fairy? You were certain that she would pay you royally for
that little tooth you lost. You were never disappointed either.

Jesus said, "Suffer the little children to come unto me, for to them belongs the Kingdom of God." Little children look at the world through the eyes of wonder and awe. Everything they behold is magnificent. They are filled with trust (until we teach them that it isn't safe to trust). They are innocent. A child comes into this world with the instinctual knowing that they will be provided for. They turn their little head and expect the nipple to sustain them with nutrition. A child expects his father and mother to take complete care of him or her, and most of the time this is how it works.

Somewhere along the way, we 'grow up' and forget that our 'Father / Mother' will provide us with what we need. Life happens, little disappointments, larger betrayals, and eventually we turn to struggle as a way of life, working hard to make ends meet. At a level of mass consciousness, we internalize a program that tells us that we have to work hard at everything—career, relationships, physical fitness, every aspect of life! When all the while, everything we desire is waiting in the etheric—ready to manifest if we will only allow it. The guideline of least expenditure of force always works, but we keep running it in the background, not unlike a computer operating system we forget is there until the system hangs up. We lose the sense of wonder and replace it with wondering.

Wondering is another face of fear. It hides the mask of doubt, and fear and doubt are the major blocks to manifesting. It is difficult, if not impossible, to see the realization of your dream if you are in doubt, wondering what is going to happen or when it might occur. When you are wondering, you are not in the present moment where conscious creation actually takes place, so you are negating your own abilities.

If you are in doubt about whether you are in wonder or wondering, here are some clues to watch for. If you are asking questions such as 'when will the money arrive?' 'Is Bob really in love with me' or 'How am I going to pay my rent on Friday?' You are wondering. If your thoughts are 'I have plenty of money, thank you' and 'Bob is the perfect partner for me at this time to assist me to learn how to love' then you are in wonder. Examine your thoughts. They will tell you the truth every time!

Wondering can be costly. For many years I have used kinesi-ology to access my protocol in the InnerSpeak process. The body doesn't lie, and since our higher selves know everything, it's the perfect tool to gain accurate information about what's going on with a person right here, right now. As I have shared, somewhere along the way I allowed myself to be duped into believing that I could use this tool to predict the future. I figured that if it worked for the present moment and since we have access to the universal subconscious, of course it would work. I fell headlong into doubt. What I didn't realize was that this questioning was delaying, even stopping my ability to create! Once I was able to break myself of this detrimental habit, I remembered wonder. I returned to trust and moved closer to heaven on earth.

When you can spend most of your time in the childlike place of wonder and awe, you will be amazed at the blessings the Universe bestows on you. Children don't judge, so they don't block the flow, and if you can emulate them, you won't block yourself either. Allow certainty to replace doubt, and you will find it so much easier to stay in the present and create peace, joy and abundance in your life.

There are several ways to heal the need to doubt and build

your trust. Let's examine some of them now:

- First, count your blessings—the things you already have in your life. When you focus on gratitude, you pull yourself into the present and release any concern about the future. Make a list of twenty things you are grateful for right now.
- Second, let go of the need to be in control—of your life, of anything! I call this "walking in surrender". The truth is you can't really control anything. It's just an illusion we have believed for aeons. Let go and "Let God…"
- Third, play the Creation Game. Close your eyes and see a blank canvas in your imagination. Paint the reality you desire on the canvas. Use as many different colors as you can think of, and make sure that every inch of the canvas is filled with the things that delight you. When you feel complete, hand the beautiful canvas to one of your Angels so that it can be given to the Universe and returned to you in an even better form than what you dreamed possible!
- Finally, have a "play date" with yourself. Go to a park this afternoon, after school is out for the day. Observe the children; watch how they relate to nature and to each other. Use what you see to help you to remember how to be a kid once more.

Chapter Twenty-Four

The Physical Piece

Your physical body is a marvelous demonstration of your capacity to create. It has capabilities that your modern medicine has yet to find or understand, abilities that in the past were considered to be magic, but that soon will be common-place for anyone with the desire to use them.

The human body is a marvelous manifesting machine. This is what it was designed to do, but there are very few biologists or doctors who will agree with that. Just think about it. The body starts off as a single cell and over a nine-month period it grows to be an eight-pound or so squirming, crying little human being. And it doesn't stop there. It continues to evolve itself year after year adding weight, height, hair and more. And it doesn't stop there either—almost every part of the body replaces itself, regen-erating new cells to replace the worn out ones—constantly. It is amazing, just from the basic physical perspective.

But if you look deeper into the lesser-known glands in the endocrine system, you will find that they perform functions of which you were totally unaware. The pituitary and pineal glands in the middle of your head actually are tiny transmitter/receivers keeping you in constant communication with the Universe. Your brain is a supercomputer, and it is generally accepted that we don't use ninety percent of its capacity. So today I am going to teach you how to use these tools to your advantage so that you can take your conscious creation skills to a totally new dimension (literally—the fifth dimension!)

The pineal and pituitary glands are vital parts of our psychic development, but they also play very critical roles in the endocrine system and everyday health and well being in the body. The hormones released directly into the bloodstream by these glands govern all aspects of growth, development, and daily physical activity. Dysfunction by any of the endocrine glands can have serious physical consequences. Energetic disturbances occur as well. A wounded pineal gland blocks our ability to communicate with our Higher Self or Source. Wounds to the pituitary prevent us from taking control of our lives, causing us to create situations of lack and resignation. Physical malfunction is itself the result of a breakdown that becomes lodged within the energy network of nodes and chakras, which we are going to talk about in a moment.

How Universal energy can stimulate the pineal and pituitary glands

Spiritual or energy healing dates back to ancient times, and is documented in many different, ancient cultures. Everything is energy, and using energy with intention to heal can have a profound effect. Even physical disease can be cured when the hidden wounds, emotional traumas, stress and inappropriate programs are released.

We have the ability to regulate pineal and pituitary function through intention and attention. Modern biological science explains this as a chemical change produced by the endocrine glands when their secretions are mixed directly into the bloodstream. Today, I offer another theory about this chemical change and how it can also be used in the process of manifestation.The chakras function as transmitters of energy from one level to another, distributing life force energy to the physical body. Each of the chakras is related to a major gland. The first chakra (base chakra) is related to the adrenal glands. The second chakra is related to ovaries in women and the prostate gland in men. The third chakra is related to the pancreas. The fourth chakra is related to the thymus gland. The fifth chakra is related to the thyroid and parathyroid glands. The sixth chakra is most often assigned to the pituitary gland and the seventh chakra to the pineal gland.

On the physical level, the seventh chakra is tied to the activity of the cerebral cortex and general nervous system functioning. In addition, the proper activation of the pineal gland/seventh chakra influences the synchronization between the left and the right hemispheres of the brain. This is the ultimate goal for all those who are both attaining the 'walking meditative' state and seeking to master the goal of conscious creation. For this chakra to be fully awakened there must first occur a balancing of body, mind and spirit. Activating the pineal and pituitary glands can create a dialog between the right and left side of your brain allowing full communication in this area, in short, an awakening. When the pineal gland/seventh chakra is activated, the sixth chakra/pituitary/third eye functions as a link between the pituitary and pineal glands.

The pineal gland

The pineal gland is cone-shaped, about the size of a pea, and is in the center of the brain in a tiny cave behind and above the pituitary gland which lies a little behind the root of the nose. The pineal gland is attached to the third ventricle of the brain. It contains a pigment similar to that in the retina of the eye and also collections of what have been called 'brain sand particles' or 'crystals.'

It has also been suggested that this gland regulates our susceptibility to light; that it has an effect upon sexuality and is related to brain growth. Beyond these facts or conjectures, investigators frankly say they know nothing, and experiments have produced little information.

It is believed that the pineal gland was, in earliest mankind, an exterior organ of physical vision, and of spiritual and psychic sight. But due to our evolutionary choices, over time passed our present two eyes began to show themselves, the pineal gland or the 'third eye', began to recede within the skull, and was covered bone and hair. It then lost its function as an organ of physical vision, but has never ceased to function as an organ of spiritual sight and insight. When you have a hunch, the pineal gland vibrates gently. It has many important hormonal functions in the body as well. Only recently have scientists uncovered its role in the aging process. It also regulates all blood pressure, body temperature, growth motor function, the reproductive system, and sleep habits. It was once considered to be a rudimentary organ and thought to have no role in human physiology.

Regulated by sunlight, and geomagnetic fields, the pineal gland plays an integral role in body cycles, controlling metabolism behavior, and physiological function. It has an intimate relationship with the pituitary gland and has a direct effect upon the adrenal glands when the body is under stress and threatened.

Non-physical pineal functions

Mystical traditions and esoteric schools have long known the pineal to be the connecting link between the physical and spiritual worlds. Adepts have always known the importance of the pineal in the initiation of psychic abilities. Most textbooks note that the pineal gland is stated by ancient philosophers to be the seat of the soul, and Descartes is quoted as saying, 'In man, soul and body touch each other only at a single point, the pineal gland in the head.'

Ancient Greeks believed the pineal gland to be our connection to the Realms of Thought. When the pineal gland awakens one feels a pressure at the base of the brain. This pressure will often be experienced when connecting to higher frequency. A head injury can also activate the Third Eye/ Pineal Gland, initiating the line of communication with the higher planes. The crown chakra reaches down until its vortex touches the pineal gland, and one's frequency is elevated from an emotional nature into awareness. The pineal and pituitary glands have a non-medical function—that of transmitter and receiver of etheric information.

The pituitary gland

The pituitary gland is about the size of a pea and is located behind the center of our forehead, between our eyes. Therefore, the sixth chakra is often called the Brow Chakra or the Third Eye. The pituitary gland is known as the master gland because it acts as a main control center that sends messages to all the other glands from its two lobes, the posterior and the anterior. The pituitary gland controls the growth of our glands and organs and regulates sexual development.

The pituitary gland has been called the 'seat of the mind'. It has two parts, or lobes. The frontal lobe regulates emotional thoughts such as poetry and music, and the posterior lobe regulates concrete thought and intellectual concepts. The function of the posterior lobe is to free ourselves from grief, and when we store wounds there, we experience fluid imbalances in the physical body, and we make decisions that create situations of 'not enough' – money, love, etc.

The function of the anterior lobe is to help us to observe, coordinate and direct. It gets wounded with memories of being controlled by someone else. Wounds here prevent us from taking control of our own lives and cause us to just give up. On the other hand, the pineal gland is known as the "seat of illumination, intuition and cosmic consciousness". The pineal gland is to the pituitary gland what intuition is to reason.

Through placing your intention and attention on the pineal and pituitary glands you will see a dramatic difference in communication in your day-to-day life. You will be more connected and aware of your own physical and mental abilities, supported by a 'knowing' that enhances your desire to create perfection for yourself. You will notice the ability to hear the 'inner' of both yourself and other people is greatly enhanced as well. Listen to this inner voice in your day-to-day life. It strengthens the 'muscle' and positively reinforces your commitment to be a higher spiritual human being. Disregard that old voice that once told you only 'they' (meaning others) can access this information and healing abilities.

Manna

I term the hormonal secretion of the active pineal gland to be manna. It has the property of the total creative ingredient, in that it can 'feed' our body, 'heal' our body, and assist in the manifestation process. It responds to our intent. When attention is placed on the pineal, manna is released. Then, with intent, you can send the manna to any area of your body to heal or feed it. In this way, the pineal gland is able to provide your daily bread, as mentioned in ancient scriptures.

Another form of manna is the energy we can request and receive from the Universe at any time. It's quite simple actually. You state (out loud preferred), "I now give to my body the energy that it requires for now and for the future and so be it," then you sit quietly and listen to your body. Your heart rate will speed up a bit as the energy flows in through your crown chakra, and will settle down when you have received what you asked for. Do this as many times during the day as you remember. You can't give yourself too much manna!

There are several ways to stimulate the pineal and pituitary glands. Due to their location inside your head, actually in the very middle of the skull on an axis formed by the temples and the front and back of the forehead, it is easy to activate them by chanting or toning. I suggest using the seed sounds of OM or AUM, which work very well. Intone these vowel sounds then close your mouth and hum the final consonant. Notice how this causes the roof of your mouth to vibrate? These vibrations stimulate the pineal and pituitary, actually waking them up! I suggest that you practice this every morning and evening, toning the sound you select seven times twice a day.

Manna meditation

Here is another way to stimulate the pineal to secrete Manna.
Let's do a little meditation:

Close your eyes and focus on your breathing. Allow yourself
to become very relaxed, letting all the concerns of the day drift
away, floating on the gentle water of a small stream. Put your
attention on the pineal gland in the middle of your head and
ask it to secrete Manna for you. Pay attention as you feel this
warm, honey-like secretion beginning to flow. Move the
Manna with your intent to any area of your body that feels
pain, stress, or just 'stuck'. Allow it to seep down your spine
and fill these areas with its peace. If there is something you
desire to create, flow the manna out to the vision of your
creation. Manna also has the property of assisting your
manifestations to move into reality, so use it liberally. When
you feel complete, thank your pineal gland for providing for
you.

Chapter Twenty Five
Shift Happens!

Now you have the tools and information to make it possible for you to create everything you have ever desired. You have received your daily bread, the manna to support you going forward. But there are just four pre-requisites that have to be kept in mind.

First, the Universe doesn't give us what we don't ask for. This works both ways—if you got it, rest assured that you "thought it up," and if you didn't get something you desired, you didn't follow the rules we've discussed!

Second, you have to participate in the equation. This means that once you set the wheels in motion by thinking of your desired result, you have to keep flowing energy into your request. Here's the best example I can give: many of us want to lose weight. What woman on the planet today is completely satisfied with her size, right? But merely thinking about losing weight doesn't generally cause the excess pounds to vanish. Healthy eating and moderate exercise bring great results every time. Another example is desiring a career change—doesn't do too much good to desire it if you never get around to creating a resume or submitting it to potential new companies.

Third, change occurs at your level of belief. If you think it can happen, it will, and if you don't believe it to be possible it will never be possible. Remember, God's answer to every prayer is 'Yes'.

Fourth, gratitude is the glue that puts it all together. That is why I always suggest that you phrase your requests on the Cosmic in the form of a gratitude statement: 'Thank you that I have already received the object of my desire, easily and in a perfect way. This or something better is mine now, and I am grateful!'

Now you have opened the door to the field of pure potential. Millions of choices lie just across the threshold, limited only by your imagination. You have become the master magician from the fables of yore. NOW you are completely in charge of your experience on the earth plane. You have cleared away the paradigms of the past and learned how to control your magic. Going forward everything you desire comes when you utter two little words:

What IF...

Beings of Now Messages

The Beings of NOW consistently bring timely messages to support us as we step into our power and build this new reality, one step at a time. Here is a selection that didn't seem to fit into the tone of this book but really did need to be included:

Today I asked the Beings of NOW why I have been feeling so disconnected - from my guides, my path and my clients. Their reply was not quite what I expected:

"This disconnection is an illusion of your own creation, Dear One. Sometimes when change is too rapid or energy too intense you think you have to pull back or risk being burned up. But that is just fear - an old belief that said that if you looked into the face of God you would be consumed by fire.

You look into the face of God every time you gaze into a mirror—or into the eyes of another human, and you are still alive, are you not?

This is illusion designed to keep you stuck in the lower vibrations... So if we told you to pull on your 'big girl panties' and get over it, would that seem too harsh? You can choose to wander in the wilderness for as long as you desire, or you can step up and step out. Your choice. Your mission will be there when you decide to do it. There is no time limit and nobody will take it away from you. It's uniquely yours."

"What we do need to discuss today is TRUST. Where you are moving when you take your next step is into trust - into certainty. It's what you requested, remember? This is why all your doubts are hanging around you like red flags, so you can see them, acknowledge their lack of existence and let them go - once and for all time."

"Did you hear the click? Do you understand what just occurred? Yesterday was an activation of a series of portals - one in the US in Arkansas, one in Bolivia and one in Mongolia. You have entered into the next phase of this Big Shift. Let's just call it Phase 2 of In-Lighten-Ment.

As these portals came online, the human species received an activation as well, expansion of your heart centers and opening of your Heart Portal, your connection to the multidimensional aspect of the New Reality.

What does this mean? Your energetic heart center in your NOW time here is now connected to the energetic heart center of each of your aspects in all other dimensions. This is an enormous step forward into the unification of your Soul back into one.

Now, if you so choose, with your attention and intention you can reach out and align with any or all of your aspects at will. Ask and it is so. In this new reality you can access via your Heart Portal all the gifts and abilities that belong to you in every dimension. The ramifications of this are infinite! No longer are you bound by the fragmentation game you created for yourselves so very long ago!

Now you can find all those gifts, abilities and things you left in other dimensions and thought you had lost - your car keys perhaps (smile). Loss was always an illusion of your own creation. It has served its purpose and it is complete.

Have fun! Play with this newness! Stay in awe and wonder, children of Light! Know that you are deeply loved and share that in every moment with each other!"

"Today we wish to discuss with you 'work' in this new reality.

For too long now humans have equated work with struggle. You have held a belief system that work was the only way you could receive prosperity. We tell you today that it is time for you to release this belief system, and we will offer a new paradigm for your consideration.

There are three parts to manifesting abundance (and none of them involves w-o-r-k).

They are:

- Understanding and claiming your power
- Service in your unique mission (which you become aware of when you claim your power)
- Aligning with and accepting prosperity in all areas of your life"

"That's it. When you establish the certainty of who you are, you become I AM. This single act places you fully into the present. In order to understand this, it will be easier if you have a clear understanding of what is 'now'. (As We are The Beings of NOW, it behooves us to share this with you!) NOW is the entirety of reality. It encompasses the past NOW, the I AM or present NOW and the future NOW. As we have told you many times before, linear time is an illusion, and once you grasp this concept, you can see more clearly how it is possible for you to reach into what you call the "future" to bring into the I AM present anything you desire. Get it? As long as what you reach for is in alignment with your purpose and is used in service to the all, this can be instantaneous, because it is fueled and supported by Source energy.

Service is best accomplished when you are open, clear and willing. When you are closed and living in the illusion of lack, fear or any other energy that is not love, you will not only be pulled off your intended direction, but you will not see the prosperity that surrounds you. It is ALWAYS there. You are all energetic symbols of the Divine. As you perceive each other, do so with an open heart and see the light that exists in all, because everyone you see is a reflection of your soul.

We have arrived at a point where you cannot afford to be confused or misshapen by old belief systems or paradigms of reality. Today is a new day on Planet Earth. As you align with the Galactic Center, Truth is streaming into each of you. Open your heart to receive this phenomenal download. You ARE connected with your Source. You are powered by the frequency of love. You are complete in every way.

And, you are respected and honored by us for your service to the One. We are in love with you!

What can we do to gain acceptance in this world? It's the big human question, isn't it? We all want to be appreciated for who we are. We want to be loved. We want to be wanted. We ask, "Can you get me?" But the underlying question is, 'Can you get YOU?'"

Acknowledgements

Many people have influenced me in the creation of this book, far too many to name, but I shall try:

Eric Hamel, the Liberator, helped me to dig deep to liberate so many wounds and free myself to move forward on my path. (www.erichamel.com)

Steve Rother, constant mentor to me and many others, has provided the encouragement we needed to speak our truth. (www.lightworker.com)

Dee Wallace, incredible Bright Light, showed me how to stand in my integrity and speak my truth (www.iamdeewallace.com)

About the Author

Jean Adrienne is a healer, teacher, breakthrough coach, lecturer and creator of quantum change. She is a graduate of The Florida State University with a BA in Psychology. She also completed The University of the South's four-year Education For Ministry program. She developed and teaches the InnerSpeak Breakthrough Process. She offers readings, coaching and clearing sessions via phone as well as in her office in Atlanta, Georgia. As an anchor writer for Sibyl Magazine and Spectrum on Lightworker.com, Jean contributes her work regularly on the Internet.

Jean Adrienne's other books - Reframe Your World: Conscious Living In The New Reality and Soul Adventures are available for purchase on her website (www.JeanAdrienne.com), Amazon.com, and in your local bookstore. She has a line of meditation CD's, the InnerSpeak Cards, and Reconnecting Soul DNA Activation Cards as well.

Soul Rocks is a fresh list that takes the search for soul and spirit mainstream. Chick-lit, young adult, cult, fashionable fiction & non-fiction with a fierce twist